METHODS IN MOLECULAR BIOLOG

Series Editor
John M. Walker
School of Life Sciences
University of Hertfordshire
Hatfield, Hertfordshire, AL10 9AB, UK

For further volumes:
http://www.springer.com/series/7651

Osteoporosis and Osteoarthritis

Second Edition

Edited by

Jennifer J. Westendorf and Andre J. van Wijnen

Mayo Clinic, Rochester, MN, USA

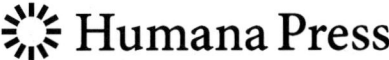

Editors
Jennifer J. Westendorf
Mayo Clinic
Rochester, MN, USA

Andre J. van Wijnen
Mayo Clinic
Rochester, MN, USA

ISSN 1064-3745   ISSN 1940-6029 (electronic)
ISBN 978-1-4939-1618-4   ISBN 978-1-4939-1619-1 (eBook)
DOI 10.1007/978-1-4939-1619-1
Springer New York Heidelberg Dordrecht London

Library of Congress Control Number: 2014949775

Humana Press is a brand of Springer
Springer is part of Springer Science+Business Media (www.springer.com)

Preface

Osteoporosis and osteoarthritis are degenerative diseases and major health problems of the twenty-first century. Osteoporosis is characterized by reduced bone mass and strength. It typically afflicts women in the sixth decade of life and men a couple of decades later. Reduced bone mass caused by the menopause, medical therapies such as corticosteroids and chemotherapy, lack of exercise, genetics, and/or environmental factors increases the risk of fractures and reduces the quality of life. Osteoarthritis is a degenerative disease that is characterized by cartilage deterioration and joint pain. It is caused by posttraumatic joint injuries or biomechanical imperfections that combined with repetitive joint motion induce wear-and-tear over time. Like osteoporosis, osteoarthritis is a debilitating disease, but it can afflict individuals at much younger ages. Together, these two diseases affect most people as they age and account for many physician visits in developed countries.

A number of advances have been made during the last few decades that enhanced detection and treatment of bone lose, but there are no proven disease-modifying therapies yet for osteoarthritis. The techniques described in this textbook are some of the most modern tools available to enhance discovery in bone and cartilage biology and promote translational research in osteoporosis and osteoarthritis. Most of the techniques in these chapters can be applied to the study of either disease, because bone formation sometimes involves a cartilage intermediate, while enhanced subchondral bone formation and osteophytes are present in osteoarthritic joints.

The goal of this textbook is to share successful protocols developed by accomplished musculoskeletal researchers. Chapters 1–5 describe methods to isolate and culture osteoblasts, osteocytes, chondrocytes, and mesenchymal progenitor cells. Methods to generate induced pluripotent stem cells are also provided. Skeletal cells have unique molecular signatures and extracellular matrices. Thus, Chapters 6–8 contain protocols to perform high-throughput methods for chromatin analysis (i.e., "ChIP-seq") in osteoblasts, identify microRNAs in human plasma for early disease detection, and execute immunohistochemistry of skeletal tissues. Mechanical loading is important for increasing bone formation, and Chapters 9 and 10 describe protocols for assessing loads on bone cells in vivo and in vitro. Chapter 11 explains a state-of-the art technique for imaging articular cartilage thickness and biochemical properties. Finally, Chapters 12–15 describe animal models to study osteoarthritis disease progression and bone healing.

We thank the authors for sharing their trusted protocols. Their time and effort in writing these chapters and producing helpful notes and illustrations are much appreciated. We also thank John Walker and Natalia van Wijnen for keeping us on schedule and helping to edit the text.

We hope these contents will inspire new research questions and accelerate therapeutic advances for the treatment of osteoporosis and osteoarthritis.

Rochester, MN, USA   *Andre J. van Wijnen*
                                                                Jennifer J. Westendorf

Contents

Contributors

RODRIGO D. ALVES • *Department of Internal Medicine, Erasmus MC, Rotterdam, The Netherlands*

NANCY A. BENKUSKY • *Department of Biochemistry, University of Wisconsin, Madison, WI, USA*

LYNDA F. BONEWALD • *Department of Oral and Craniofacial Sciences, School of Dentistry, University of Missouri-Kansas City, Kansas City, MO, USA*

JUN CHANG • *Research Division, Hospital for Special Surgery, New York, NY, USA*

JONATHAN COICO • *Tissue Engineering Regeneration and Repair Program, Research Division, Hospital for Special Surgery, New York, NY, USA*

KIRSTY L. CULLY • *Tissue Engineering Regeneration and Repair Program, Research Division, Hospital for Special Surgery, New York, NY, USA*

ELIZABETH N. DELASSUS • *Musculoskeletal Research Center, Histology and Morphometry Core, Department of Orthopedics, Washington University School of Medicine, St. Louis, MO, USA*

DAVID R. DEYLE • *Department of Medical Genetics, Mayo Clinic, Rochester, MN, USA*

CECILIA L. DRAGOMIR • *Tissue Engineering Regeneration and Repair Program, Research Division, Hospital for Special Surgery, New York, NY, USA*

HICHAM DRISSI • *New England Musculoskeletal Institute, University of Connecticut Health Center, Farmington, CT, USA*

BRAM C. VAN DER EERDEN • *Department of Internal Medicine, Erasmus MC, Rotterdam, The Netherlands*

GABRIEL L. GALEA • *School of Veterinary Sciences, University of Bristol, Bristol, UK*

MARY B. GOLDRING • *Tissue Engineering Regeneration and Repair Program, Research Division, Hospital for Special Surgery, New York, NY, USA*

ROBERT E. GULDBERG • *George W. Woodruff School of Mechanical Engineering, Georgia Institute of Technology, Atlanta, GA, USA; Parker H. Petit Institute for Bioengineering & Bioscience, Georgia Institute of Technology, Atlanta, GA, USA*

DONNA HOAK • *Department of Orthopaedics, University of Rochester Medical Center, Rochester, NY, USA*

CRYSTAL IDLEBURG • *Musculoskeletal Research Center, Histology and Morphometry Core, Department of Orthopedics, Washington University School of Medicine, St. Louis, MO, USA*

WILFRED F. VAN IJCKEN • *Erasmus Center for Biomics, Erasmus MC, Rotterdam, The Netherlands*

HEE-JEONG IM • *Departments of Biochemistry, Orthopedic Surgery and Medicine, Section of Rheumatology, Rush University Medical Center, Chicago, IL, USA*

JENNIFER H. JONASON • *Department of Orthopaedics, University of Rochester Medical Center, Rochester, NY, USA*

MARCEL KARPERIEN • *Department of Developmental Bioengineering, MIRA Institute for Biomedical Technology and Technical Medicine, University of Twente, Enschede, The Netherlands*

CHRISTEL E. KOCKX • *Erasmus Center for Biomics, Erasmus MC, Rotterdam, The Netherlands*

JEFFREY S. KROIN • *Department of Anesthesiology, Rush University Medical Center, Chicago, IL, USA*

JOHANNES P. VAN LEEUWEN • *Department of Internal Medicine, Erasmus MC, Rotterdam, The Netherlands*

ANGELA S.P. LIN • *George W. Woodruff School of Mechanical Engineering, Georgia Institute of Technology, Atlanta, GA, USA; Parker H. Petit Institute for Bioengineering and Bioscience, Georgia Institute of Technology, Atlanta, GA, USA*

MEGHAN E. MCGEE-LAWRENCE • *Department of Cellular Biology and Anatomy, Georgia Regents University, GA, USA; Department of Orthopedics, Mayo Clinic, Rochester, MN, USA*

KATHERINE M. MELVILLE • *Department of Biomedical Engineering, Cornell University, Ithaca, NY, USA; Sibley School of Mechanical and Aerospace Engineering, Cornell University, Ithaca, NY, USA*

MARJOLEIN C.H. VAN DER MEULEN • *Sibley School of Mechanical and Aerospace Engineering, Cornell University, Ithaca, NY, USA; Research Division, Hospital for Special Surgery, New York, NY, USA*

MARK B. MEYER • *Department of Biochemistry, University of Wisconsin, Madison, WI, USA*

DEBORAH V. NOVACK • *Musculoskeletal Research Center, Histology and Morphometry Core, Departments of Medicine and Pathology, Washington University School of Medicine, St. Louis, MO, USA*

REGIS J. O'KEEFE • *Department of Orthopaedics, University of Rochester Medical Center, Rochester, NY, USA*

MIGUEL OTERO • *Tissue Engineering Regeneration and Repair Program, Research Division, Hospital for Special Surgery, New York, NY, USA*

ZELIHA OZGUR • *Erasmus Center for Biomics, Erasmus MC, Rotterdam, The Netherlands*

DAVID N. PAGLIA • *New England Musculoskeletal Institute, University of Connecticut Health Center, Farmington, CT, USA*

JEROEN VAN DE PEPPEL • *Department of Internal Medicine, Erasmus MC, Rotterdam, The Netherlands*

MARGARET J. PIEL • *Comparative Medicine Consultants, Chicago, IL, USA*

J. WESLEY PIKE • *Department of Biochemistry, University of Wisconsin, Madison, WI, USA*

DARREN A. PLUMB • *Breakthrough Breast Cancer Research Unit, King's College London School of Medicine, Guy's Hospital, London, UK*

JANINE N. POST • *Department of Developmental Bioengineering, MIRA Institute for Biomedical Technology and Technical Medicine, University of Twente, Enschede, The Netherlands*

JOANNA S. PRICE • *School of Veterinary Sciences, University of Bristol, Bristol, UK*

LING QIN • *Department of Orthopaedic Surgery, Perelman School of Medicine, University of Pennsylvania, Philadelphia, PA, USA*

DAVID F. RAZIDLO • *Mayo Clinic, Rochester, MN, USA*

ALEXANDER G. ROBLING • *Department of Anatomy and Cell Biology, Indiana University School of Medicine, Indianapolis, IN, USA; Department of Biomedical Engineering, Indiana University School of Medicine, Indianapolis, IN, USA*

GIULIANA E. SALAZAR-NORATTO • *Wallace H. Coulter Department of Biomedical Engineering, Georgia Institute of Technology, Atlanta, GA, USA*

MARIJKE SCHREUDERS-KOEDAM • *Department of Internal Medicine, Erasmus MC, Rotterdam, The Netherlands*

VALERIE A. SICLARI • *Department of Orthopaedic Surgery, Perelman School of Medicine, University of Pennsylvania, Philadelphia, PA, USA*

AMBER RATH STERN • *Department of Oral and Craniofacial Sciences, School of Dentistry, University of Missouri-Kansas City, Kansas City, MO, USA*

ELISABETH B. WONDIMU • *Research Division, Hospital for Special Surgery, New York, NY, USA*

LING WU • *Department of Orthopaedic Surgery, Orthopedic Hospital Research Center, David Geffen School of Medicine, University of California at Los Angeles, Los Angeles, CA, USA*

JI ZHU • *Department of Orthopaedic Surgery, Perelman School of Medicine, University of Pennsylvania, Philadelphia, PA, USA*

Part I

Cell Biology

Chapter 1

Isolation of Osteocytes from Mature and Aged Murine Bone

Amber Rath Stern and Lynda F. Bonewald

Abstract

Osteocytes are thought to be the mechanosensors of bone by sensing mechanical loads imposed upon the bone and transmitting these signals to the other bone cells to initiate bone modeling and remodeling. The location of osteocytes deep within bone is ideal for their function. However, this location makes the study of osteocytes in vivo technically difficult. There are several methods for obtaining and culturing primary osteocytes for in vitro experiments and ex vivo observation. In this chapter, several proven methods are discussed including the isolation of avian osteocytes from chicks and osteocytes from calvaria and long bones of young mice. A detailed protocol for the isolation of osteocytes from hypermineralized bone of mature and aged animals is provided.

Key words Osteocyte, Isolation, Age, Culture, Collagenase, Mice

1 Introduction

Osteocytes are the most abundant of the bone cells and are recently found to be multifunctional [1, 2]. They serve as orchestrators of bone remodeling and regulators of mineral homeostasis. They are the mechanosensors of bone, sensing imposed bone loads, and translating these mechanical signals into biological signals of bone modeling and remodeling. They are housed in cave-like voids within the bone called lacunae. Their location deep within the mineralized bone matrix is ideal for their cellular functions, but makes their observation and study difficult. Methods to isolate these bone matrix-embedded cells have been developed throughout the years and vary by the species, state, and extent of mineralization of the bone.

In 1992, the group of Peter Nijweide was the first to describe the isolation of osteocytes from 18-day-old chick embryos. Their approach yielded a relatively pure population of osteocytes based on morphology [3]. In 1995, Kumegawa and colleagues published a method for isolating primary avian osteocytes from the parietal

Jennifer J. Westendorf and Andre J. van Wijnen (eds.), *Osteoporosis and Osteoarthritis*, Methods in Molecular Biology, vol. 1226, DOI 10.1007/978-1-4939-1619-1_1, © Springer Science+Business Media New York 2015

bones of 16-day-old chick embryos [4]. Osteocyte morphology and possible dedifferentiation into osteoblasts was noted in this study. The method proved reproducible and useful in isolating primary avian osteocytes for study by other researchers [5–12]. The bones isolated from the chick embryos are essentially paper thin and not yet mineralized. The parietal bone is flexible and easy to digest, making the isolation of avian embryonic osteocytes rather quick and straightforward. However, the drawbacks of this initial method were that the primary osteocytes are very young themselves because they were isolated from embryonic bone, and they were avian, not mammalian. The need to develop isolation methods for osteocytes from other species was apparent.

A method for isolating primary osteocytes from the calvaria of neonatal rats was described in 1995 [13]. Mikuni-Takagaki et al. characterized the osteoblast–osteocyte lineage by describing the subpopulations of isolated cells. These methods were utilized in several subsequent publications on the investigation of the mechanotransduction of osteocytes [14–16]. These studies showed that the various populations of isolated bone cells responded to mechanical strain in different manners and at different magnitudes, providing insight into the highly strain-responsive nature of osteocytes. Other researchers have also utilized this method in their studies of primary neonatal rat calvaria osteocytes [17].

Calvaria from young chicks and neonatal rats are all very thin and easily processed using sequential collagenase digestions and calcium chelation with EDTA (ethylenediaminetetraacetic acid). The rationale for these sequential steps is that removal of mineral exposes collagen fibers that if digested will release cells embedded in mineralized tissue. Studies utilizing these primary osteocytes can provide insight into the behavior of osteocytes during early development but are not suitable for the study of osteocytes from skeletally mature bone, and do not allow the comparison between primary osteocytes isolated from animals of different ages, species, and genotypes. The calvaria are also not bones that are typically mechanically loaded longitudinally during everyday activity and regularly modeled and remodeled, such as the long bones (femurs, humeri, and tibiae). Methods for isolating calvarial osteocytes have also been adapted and applied to the isolation of osteocytes from neonatal and very young murine long bones with success, and were even utilized in the creation of several osteocyte-like cell lines from mice of 2–3 months of age [18–20]. This method was used to compare osteoblast and osteocyte function and gene expression in several studies [21–23].

To study the effects of age on osteocytes and osteocytes isolated from high bone mass mice, a method for isolating primary osteocytes from hypermineralized bone was still needed. When the methods for isolating primary osteocytes from hypomineralized bone such as young calvaria and long bones were employed for hypermineralized bone, they produced a very low yield rate mainly yielding only the surface cells and shallowly embedded osteocytes. When characterized, the populations of cells were mixed with considerable variation from isolation to isolation. We recently published a method for isolating osteocytes from hypermineralized bone utilizing nine sequential collagenase and EDTA treatments. It is similar to previous methods, but key differences are that, the periosteum was removed, and a tissue homogenizer was employed prior to the final digestion [24]. This method has been utilized by several laboratories to isolate primary osteocytes from mature (4–6 months) and aged (22–24 months) murine bone [25, 26].

2 Materials

This technique facilitates the isolation of osteocytes from skeletally mature bone (older than 3–4 months) to aged bone (22–24 months), and was originally published in *Biotechniques* [24]. The early digestions (where noted) can also be used for obtaining primary osteoblasts. Prior to starting the isolation, several solutions and media must be prepared.

1. Collagenase Solution: Dissolve 300 active units/mL of collagenase type IA (Sigma-Aldrich, St. Lewis, MO) in α–minimal essential medium (αMEM). 50 mL is adequate for an isolation from one or two mice (*see* **Note 1**).

2. EDTA Solution: Prepare the 5 mM ethylenediaminetetraacetic acid tetrasodium salt dehydrate (EDTA) solution in magnesium- and calcium-free Dulbecco's Phosphate-Buffered Solution (DPBS) with 1 % bovine serum albumin. Bring to a neutral pH of 7.4 by adding HCl. 30 mL is adequate for osteocyte isolation from one or two mice (*see* **Note 2**).

3. Primary Bone Cell Culture Medium: On the day before the isolation, supplement α–minimal essential medium (αMEM) with 5 % heat-inactivated fetal bovine serum (FBS), 5 % heat-inactivated calf serum (CS), and 1 % penicillin and streptomycin (PS). This culture medium is chosen based on the culture of the MLO-Y4 osteocyte cell line [19]. Store at 4 °C.

4. Collagen-Coated Plates: On the day before the isolation and in a sterile tissue culture hood, dilute sterile collagen in *previously filter sterilized 0.02 M acetic acid* to final concentration of *0.15 mg/mL* (*see* **Note 3**). Generally use, 8 mL for coating a 100 mm dish. Coat plates for 1 h at room temperature. Tilt to remove excess collagen and save. This solution can be reused approximately 6 times and should be kept at 4 °C. To use plates immediately, it is best to rinse the plate with PBS to remove residual acid; otherwise dry the plates for 1 h (without rinsing with PBS) with the lids off before storing at 4 °C.

5. Surgical instruments to dissect and mince bones: forceps, surgical scissors, and scalpels.

6. 25-, and/or 27-G needles and 1 mL syringes.

7. 100 % ethanol.

8. 70 % ethanol.

9. Hank's balanced salt solution (HBSS) calcium and magnesium-free.

10. α–minimal essential medium (αMEM).

11. Heat-inactivated fetal bovine serum (FBS).

12. Penicillin and streptomycin.

13. Gentamicin (optional).

14. 6-well petri dishes (non-TC treated).

15. 100 mm petri dishes (non-TC treated).

16. Shaker in incubator.

17. Tissue homogenizer (Medimachine (BD Biosciences, San Jose, CA)) with a stainless steel mincing screen with a pore size of 50 μm).

3   Methods

This protocol takes approximately 10–12 h from the time the mice are sacrificed to the time that the bone particles are plated. The length of time depends on the number of mice used and familiarity of the researchers with the protocol.

1. Aseptically dissect the long bones (femurs, tibiae, and humeri) from the mice using surgical scissors or scalpel. Be sure not to break any of the bones at this point and also try to keep the abdomen intact during the dissection to reduce contamination potential (*see* **Note 4**).

2. After dissection of bones and removal of as much soft tissue as possible, place them in 100 mm petri dishes containing αMEM with 10 % penicillin and streptomycin (and gentamicin (25 μg/mL)—optional) (*see* **Note 4**).

3. Remove any remaining muscle and connective tissue from the bones and scrape away the periosteum using a scalpel (*see* **Note 4**).

4. Wash the bones in sequential dishes/wells of a six-well plate filled with αMEM + 10 % penicillin and streptomycin to remove fur and other contaminants.

5. Place bones in a 100 mm petri dishes with fresh αMEM with 10 % penicillin and streptomycin (and gentamicin (25 μg/mL) —optional).

6. Cut off the bone epiphyses and flush the marrow out using a needle and syringe.

7. Wash the hollowed bone pieces again in αMEM with 10 % penicillin and streptomycin (and gentamicin (25 μg/mL) —optional).

8. Cut the bones in half lengthwise and then cut into 1–2 mm lengths using a scalpel.

9. As the bone pieces are cut place in HBSS for a brief wash.

10. Collagenase Treatment 1: Incubate the bone pieces in warmed collagenase solution for 25 min (*see* **Note 5**).

11. Aspirate the solution and keep for cell plating (if interested in Digest 1 cells) (*see* **Notes 6** and **7**).

12. Wash the bone pieces with HBSS three times with 5 mL each, each time adding the HBSS rinse to the aspirated solution for cell plating.

13. Pellet, resuspend, and plate the cells on collagen-coated plates using the primary bone cell culture medium.

14. Collagenase Treatment 2: Repeat **steps 10–13**.

15. Collagenase Treatment 3: Repeat **steps 10–13**, again. Combine cells with those from **step 14** (*see* **Note 8**).

16. EDTA Treatment 1: Incubate the bone pieces in warmed EDTA solution for 25 min (*see* **Note 5**).

17. Aspirate the solution and keep for cell plating (if interested in Digest 4 cells) (*see* **Notes 6** and **7**).

18. Repeat **steps 12** and **13**.

19. Collagenase Treatment 4: Incubate the bone pieces in warmed collagenase solution for 25 min (*see* **Note 5**).

20. Aspirate the solution and keep for cell plating (if interested in Digest 5 cells) (*see* **Notes 6** and **7**).

21. Repeat **steps 12** and **13** (*see* **Note 8**).

22. EDTA Treatment 2: Incubate the bone pieces in warmed EDTA solution for 25 min (*see* **Note 5**).

23. Aspirate the solution and keep for cell plating (if interested in Digest 6 cells) (*see* **Notes 6** and **7**).

24. Repeat **steps 12** and **13** (*see* **Note 9**).

25. Collagenase Treatment 5: Incubate the bone pieces in warmed collagenase solution for 25 min (*see* **Note 5**).

26. Aspirate the solution and keep for cell plating (if interested in Digest 7 cells) (*see* **Notes 6** and **7**).

27. Repeat **steps 12** and **13** (*see* **Note 10**).

28. EDTA Treatment 3: Incubate the bone pieces in warmed EDTA solution for 25 min (*see* **Note 5**).

29. Aspirate the solution and keep for cell plating (if interested in Digest 8 cells) (*see* **Notes 6** and **7**).

30. Repeat **steps 12** and **13** (*see* **Note 11**).

31. Collagenase Treatment 6: Incubate the bone pieces in warmed collagenase solution for 25 min (*see* **Note 5**).

32. Aspirate the solution and keep for cell plating (*see* **Notes 6** and **7**).

33. Repeat **steps 12** and **13** (*see* **Note 12**).

34. Mince the bone pieces in αMEM utilizing a tissue homogenizer.

35. Directly plate the resulting suspension of bone particles in αMEM on collagen-coated plates adding additional primary bone cell culture medium if needed *(see* **Note 13**).

4   Notes

1. The collagenase solution must be prepared fresh the morning of the isolation.

2. The EDTA solution can be prepared the day before the isolation and stored at 4 °C.

3. Use a chilled pipet so the collagen doesn't stick.

4. Steps one and two can be conducted on a lab bench. **Steps 3–35** should be performed in a sterile laminar flow hood.

5. 8 mL of solution per well in a six-well plate works well for the long bones from 1 to 2 mice.

6. The issue of maintaining cell density is quite crucial for the cell attachment and survival of the later digests. It is recommended for an isolation using 1–2 mature mice where it is desired to plate each digest individually, one should use a 6-well plate format. If similar digests are combined together, digests 7–9 for example, one should use a 100 mm dish format. The bone particles derived from 1 to 2 mature mice can be split between two wells of a 6-well plate.

7. Cells will be immediately visible in digests 1–9 (for cell counting and trypan blue staining) and should attach to the plate within 24–48 h. These will be primarily surface cells such as fibroblasts and osteoblasts.

8. These will be primarily osteoblastic cells.

9. These will be a mix of osteoblastic and osteocytic cells.

10. These will be primarily osteoblastic and osteocytic cells. Each subsequent serial digest will yield a greater percentage of osteocytic cells.

11. These will be primarily osteocytic cells.

12. At this point, the bone pieces can also be used for isolation of osteocyte mRNA as described previously [27]).

13. Do not disturb the bone particle cultures for at least 48 h. Moving the dish will cause movement of the bone particles and therefore hinder the attachment of the osteocytes. It is recommended to leave the bone particles for as long as possible, adding additional primary bone cell medium to the dishes at 72 h, and changing to fresh medium at 4 or 5 days post culture. It is recommended to use the osteocytic cultures for experimental purposes before day 7 as that is when they were characterized in the *BioTechniques* manuscript [24]. Prolonged culture will otherwise lead to dedifferentiation/loss of phenotype or an overgrowth of the cultures by any contaminating fibro- or osteoblasts.

References

1. Bonewald LF (2011) The amazing osteocyte. J Bone Miner Res 26:229–238

2. Dallas SL, Prideaux M, Bonewald LF (2013) The osteocyte: an endocrine cell and more. Endocr Rev 34:658–690

3. van der Plas A, Nijweide PJ (1992) Isolation and purification of osteocytes. J Bone Miner Res 7:389–396

4. Tanaka K, Matsuo T, Ohta M et al (1995) Time-lapse microcinematography of osteocytes. Miner Electrolyte Metab 21:189–192

5. Aarden EM, Nijweide PJ, van der Plas A et al (1996) Adhesive properties of isolated chick osteocytes in vitro. Bone 18:305–313

6. Ajubi NE, Klein-Nulend J, Nijweide PJ et al (1996) Pulsating fluid flow increases prostaglandin production by cultured chicken osteocytes–a cytoskeleton-dependent process. Biochem Biophys Res Commun 225:62–68

7. Kamioka H, Honjo T, Takano-Yamamoto T (2001) A three-dimensional distribution of osteocyte processes revealed by the combination of confocal laser scanning microscopy and differential interference contrast microscopy. Bone 28:145–149

8. Kamioka H, Ishihara Y, Ris H et al (2007) Primary cultures of chick osteocytes retain functional gap junctions between osteocytes and between osteocytes and osteoblasts. Microsc Microanal 13:108–117

9. Kamioka H, Sugawara Y, Murshid SA et al (2006) Fluid shear stress induces less calcium response in a single primary osteocyte than in a single osteoblast: implication of different focal adhesion formation. J Bone Miner Res 21:1012–1021

10. Klein-Nulend J, Semeins CM, Ajubi NE et al (1995) Pulsating fluid flow increases nitric oxide (NO) synthesis by osteocytes but not periosteal fibroblasts–correlation with prostaglandin upregulation. Biochem Biophys Res Commun 217:640–648

11. Klein-Nulend J, van der Plas A, Semeins CM et al (1995) Sensitivity of osteocytes to biomechanical stress in vitro. FASEB J 9: 441–445

12. Westbroek I, Ajubi NE, Alblas MJ et al (2000) Differential stimulation of prostaglandin G/H synthase-2 in osteocytes and other osteogenic cells by pulsating fluid flow. Biochem Biophys Res Commun 268:414–419

13. Mikuni-Takagaki Y, Kakai Y, Satoyoshi M et al (1995) Matrix mineralization and the differentiation of osteocyte-like cells in culture. J Bone Miner Res 10:231–242

14. Kawata A, Mikuni-Takagaki Y (1998) Mechanotransduction in stretched osteocytes–temporal expression of immediate early and other genes. Biochem Biophys Res Commun 246:404–408

15. Mikuni-Takagaki Y (1999) Mechanical responses and signal transduction pathways in stretched osteocytes. J Bone Miner Metab 17: 57–60

16. Mikuni-Takagaki Y, Suzuki Y, Kawase T et al (1996) Distinct responses of different populations of bone cells to mechanical stress. Endocrinology 137:2028–2035

17. Gu G, Hentunen TA, Nars M et al (2005) Estrogen protects primary osteocytes against glucocorticoid-induced apoptosis. Apoptosis 10:583–595

18. Kato Y, Boskey A, Spevak L et al (2001) Establishment of an osteoid preosteocyte-like cell MLO-A5 that spontaneously mineralizes in culture. J Bone Miner Res 16:1622–1633

19. Kato Y, Windle JJ, Koop BA et al (1997) Establishment of an osteocyte-like cell line, MLO-Y4. J Bone Miner Res 12:2014–2023

20. Woo SM, Rosser J, Dusevich V et al (2011) Cell line IDG-SW3 replicates osteoblast-to-late-osteocyte differentiation in vitro and accelerates bone formation in vivo. J Bone Miner Res 26:2634–2646

21. Zhao S, Zhang YK, Harris S et al (2002) MLO-Y4 osteocyte-like cells support osteoclast formation and activation. J Bone Miner Res 17:2068–2079

22. Kramer I, Halleux C, Keller H et al (2010) Osteocyte Wnt/beta-catenin signaling is required for normal bone homeostasis. Mol Cell Biol 30:3071–3085

23. Nakashima T, Hayashi M, Fukunaga T et al (2011) Evidence for osteocyte regulation of bone homeostasis through RANKL expression. Nat Med 17:1231–1234

24. Stern AR, Stern MM, Van Dyke ME et al (2012) Isolation and culture of primary osteocytes from the long bones of skeletally mature and aged mice. BioTechniques 52:361–373

25. Jahn K, Lara-Castillo N, Brotto L et al (2012) Skeletal muscle secreted factors prevent glucocorticoid-induced osteocyte apoptosis through activation of beta-catenin. Eur Cell Mater 24:197–209

26. Kalajzic I, Matthews BG, Torreggiani E et al (2013) In vitro and in vivo approaches to study osteocyte biology. Bone 54:296–306

27. Qing H, Ardeshirpour L, Pajevic PD et al (2012) Demonstration of osteocytic perilacunar/canalicular remodeling in mice during lactation. J Bone Miner Res 27:1018–1029

Chapter 2

Primary Murine Growth Plate and Articular Chondrocyte Isolation and Cell Culture

Jennifer H. Jonason, Donna Hoak, and Regis J. O'Keefe

Abstract

The ability to isolate primary chondrocytes from wild-type and genetically altered mice has provided tremendous advances in the understanding of signaling networks that regulate chondrocytes in health and disease. Isolation of chondrocytes from both growth plate tissues and articular cartilage has been challenging due to the cells being embedded within a highly organized tissue matrix. Here we describe highly reproducible methods for the isolation of pure populations of growth plate chondrocytes from the murine sternum and ribs and articular chondrocytes from the knee joint.

Key words Articular chondrocyte, Growth plate chondrocyte, Cell isolation, Articular cartilage, Growth plate cartilage, Cell culture, Tissue digestion

1 Introduction

Hyaline cartilage is a complex structure that is composed primarily of type II collagen with the addition of a number of minor collagens including IX and XI [1]. Hyaline cartilage also contains aggregating proteoglycans and other noncollagen glycoproteins [2]. Skeletal growth and development, joint formation and maintenance of articular cartilage, and bone regeneration all require coordination of a highly integrated network of signals in chondrocytes to produce and maintain cartilage tissues [3]. The ability to isolate primary chondrocytes from wild-type and genetically altered mice has provided tremendous advances in the understanding of signaling networks that regulate chondrocytes in health and disease.

While closely related, chondrocytes in the growth plate and in the articular cartilage have unique functions and behaviors. Growth plate chondrocytes are metabolically active cells that undergo a highly coordinated sequence of events that include proliferation followed by a maturation process that results in cell hypertrophy and secretion of a calcified matrix that provides a template for bone formation [3]. Fully differentiated growth plate chondrocytes

Jennifer J. Westendorf and Andre J. van Wijnen (eds.), *Osteoporosis and Osteoarthritis*, Methods in Molecular Biology, vol. 1226, DOI 10.1007/978-1-4939-1619-1_2, © Springer Science+Business Media New York 2015

provide signals for vascular ingrowth into the calcified cartilage and undergo apoptosis [4]. These cells have a high capacity for regeneration and are phenotypically similar to the chondrocyte populations involved in fracture repair [5].

In contrast, articular chondrocytes rarely proliferate in vivo and have minimal capacity for tissue regeneration [6]. Articular chondrocytes secrete and maintain a highly organized matrix meant to last the lifetime of the organism [7, 8]. Articular cartilage has extraordinary mechanical properties that provide high compressive and tensile strength and a lubricated surface that enables near frictionless gliding of opposing joint surfaces [2, 7].

Since both articular and growth plate chondrocytes are located within highly organized matrices composed of collagens, glycoproteins, and noncollagen proteins, isolation of each of these cell populations is challenging. We will provide insights into the unique procedures to isolate each of these populations.

2   Materials

2.1   Primary Murine Costal Chondrocyte Isolation

1. Neonatal mice from postnatal age (P) 2–4 days (*see* **Note 1**).
2. 70 % Ethanol.
3. Bone cutting scissors, dissection scissors, and standard forceps with blunt, serrated ends. These should be cleaned well with 70 % ethanol prior to use.
4. Sterile 10 cm petri dishes.
5. Sterile 70 μm cell strainers.
6. Sterile 50 ml polypropylene centrifuge tubes.
7. Sterile 1× Phosphate-buffered saline (PBS), pH 7.4.
8. *Pronase solution*: Dissolve Pronase (Roche) to a final concentration of 2 mg/ml in 1× PBS supplemented with 100 U/ml Penicillin and 100 U/ml Streptomycin. Make fresh and filter sterilize through a 0.2 μm filter.
9. *Collagenase D solution*: Dissolve Collagenase D (Roche) to a final concentration of 3 mg/ml in Dulbecco's modified Eagle's medium (DMEM) supplemented with 100 U/ml Penicillin and 100 μg/ml Streptomycin. Make fresh and filter sterilize through a 0.2 μm filter.
10. *Complete culture medium*: DMEM supplemented with 10 % FBS (do not heat-inactivate), 100 U/ml Penicillin and 100 μg/ml Streptomycin.

2.2   Plating and Culture of Primary Murine Costal Chondrocytes

1. Hemacytometer or automated cell counter.
2. *Complete culture medium*: DMEM supplemented with 10 % FBS (do not heat-inactivate), 100 U/ml Penicillin and 100 μg/ml Streptomycin.

3. Tissue culture-treated polystyrene multiwell plates.

4. *Chondrocyte maturation medium*: Complete culture medium supplemented with 50 µg/ml ascorbic acid and 10 mM β-glycerophosphate (*see* **Note 2**).

2.3   Isolation and Culture of Primary Murine Articular Chondrocytes

1. Mice postnatal age (P) 21–28 days.

2. 70 % Ethanol.

3. Dissection scissors and standard forceps with blunt, serrated ends. These should be cleaned well with 70 % ethanol prior to use.

4. Sterile scalpels.

5. Sterile 10 cm petri dishes.

6. Sterile 70 µm cell strainers.

7. Sterile 50 ml polypropylene centrifuge tubes.

8. Sterile 1× Phosphate-buffered saline (PBS), pH 7.4.

9. *Collagenase D solutions*: Dissolve Collagenase D (Roche) to a final concentration of either 3 mg/ml or 5 mg/ml in Dulbecco's modified Eagle's medium (DMEM) supplemented with 100 U/ml Penicillin and 100 µg/ml Streptomycin. Make fresh and filter sterilize through a 0.2 µm filter.

10. *Complete culture medium*: DMEM supplemented with 10 % FBS (do not heat-inactivate), 100 U/ml Penicillin and 100 µg/ml Streptomycin.

11. Tissue culture-treated polystyrene plates.

3   Methods

3.1   Primary Murine Costal Chondrocyte Isolation

1. Euthanize neonatal mice via an approved IACUC method and proceed immediately with the protocol to avoid loss of cell viability.

2. From this point forward, all steps should be carried out in a Class II biological safety cabinet using sterile technique.

3. Douse the body in 70 % ethanol and decapitate with bone cutting scissors. Place the body in a sterile petri dish containing cold 1× PBS positioned on ice.

4. Harvest the anterior rib cage and sternum en bloc. To do so, first remove the forelimbs and cut below the thoracic cage exposing the viscera. Remove the lower viscera, diaphragm, and upper viscera. Remove the skin. Cut parallel to one side of the vertebral column detaching all ribs from the column. Grasping the vertebral column with forceps, gently remove excess soft tissue from dorsal and ventral sides of the ribs and sternum. Cut along the other side of the vertebral column and

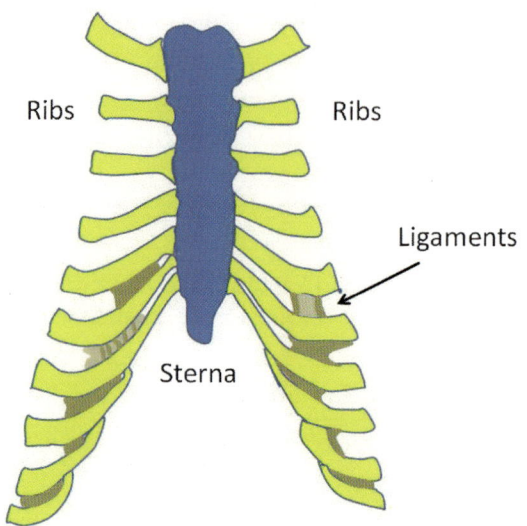

Fig. 1 Schematic mouse sterna and ribs

deposit the harvested rib cage and sternum into a 50 ml conical tube containing cold 1× PBS on ice (Fig. 1; *see* **Note 3**).

5. Carefully decant the PBS and add 15 ml of the 2 mg/ml Pronase solution. Cap the tube tightly and place in a 37 °C shaking water bath set at 70–80 rpm for 60 min (*see* **Note 4**).

6. Remove the conical tube from the water bath and spray liberally with 70 % ethanol before reentering the biological safety cabinet.

7. Carefully decant the Pronase solution and wash the sterna and ribs three times with 1× PBS. When washing, fill the conical tube with PBS, cap the tube, and swirl the tube aggressively to liberate the soft tissue. Sterna and ribs will settle on the bottom while soft tissue will float near the top. Decant the PBS and floating soft tissue.

8. Add 15 ml of the 3 mg/ml Collagenase D solution. Incubate at 37 °C in a humidified cell culture incubator for 1.5 h with a loosened lid. Agitate the tissue every 30 min to ensure adequate digestion (*see* **Note 5**).

9. Decant the Collagenase D solution. Wash sterna and ribs with 1× PBS as described in **step 6** a minimum of three times or as necessary to remove all remaining soft tissue (*see* **Note 6**).

10. Add 15 ml of the 5 mg/ml Collagenase D solution and pour ribs and sterna suspension into a sterile petri dish. Incubate at 37 °C in a humidified cell culture incubator for 3–5 h, swirling the dish every hour to encourage dissociation of the cells (*see* **Note 7**).

11. Pipette contents of the petri dish up and down a few times to break up any remaining clusters of cells and dispense over a 70 μm cell strainer positioned over a 50 ml conical tube.

12. Pellet the cells by centrifugation. Remove the Collagenase D solution by aspiration.

13. Wash the cells once in 10 ml complete culture medium to remove any residual Collagenase D solution.

14. Pellet the cells and resuspend in 10 ml complete culture medium.

3.2 Plating and Culture of Primary Murine Costal Chondrocytes

1. Determine the number of cells in the cell suspension by counting with a hemacytometer or automated cell counter.

2. Bring the cell suspension to the desired concentration with additional culture medium and plate cells at high density in the appropriate format for the desired downstream applications (*see* **Note 8**).

3. Place the plates in a humidified cell culture incubator at 37 °C with 5 % CO_2 to allow the cells to adhere to the plate.

4. If culturing for in vitro maturation assays, allow the cells to reach to confluence prior to the addition of chondrocyte maturation medium. Change this medium every 2–3 days until the desired time point of harvest.

3.3 Isolation and Culture of Primary Murine Articular Chondrocytes

1. Euthanize postnatal mice via an approved IACUC method and proceed immediately with the protocol to avoid loss of cell viability.

2. Clean fur and skin with 70 % Ethanol. Remove skin and soft tissues from the hindlimbs and dislocate the femoral head from the acetabulum. Remove the articular cartilage cap from the femoral head using blunt-ended forceps. Disarticulate the femur and tibia and place them in a petri dish containing cold 1× PBS. Use a scalpel to remove the articular cartilage from the femoral condyles and tibial plateau (Fig. 2; *see* **Note 9**).

3. Collect all articular cartilage pieces in a 50 ml conical tube containing cold 1× PBS on ice. Carefully decant the PBS and wash the cartilage three times with additional 1× PBS. When washing, fill the conical tube with PBS, cap the tube, and swirl the tube aggressively. Cartilage will settle on the bottom.

4. Add 15 ml of the 3 mg/ml Collagenase D solution and pour the cartilage suspension into a sterile petri dish. Incubate at 37 ° C in a humidified cell culture incubator overnight.

5. Pipette contents of the petri dish up and down a few times to liberate cells from the cartilage pieces and dispense over a 70 μm cell strainer positioned over a 50 ml conical tube.

6. Pellet the cells by centrifugation.

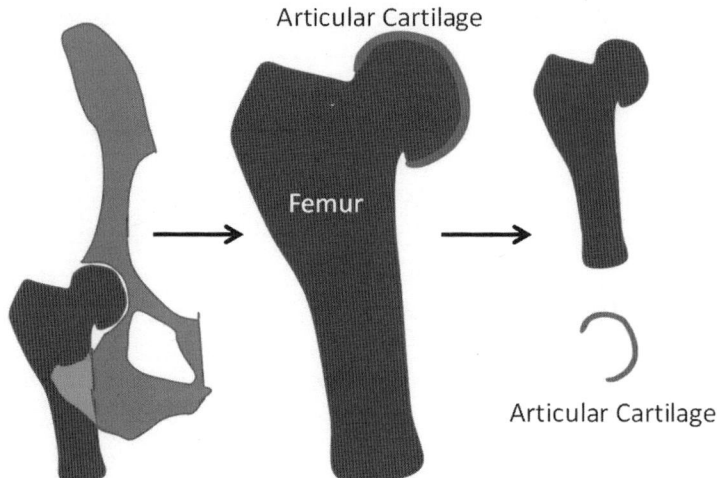

Fig. 2 Schematic of mouse femur and pelvis, proximal femur, and femur and isolated articular cartilage

7. Remove the Collagenase D solution by aspiration.

8. Add 10 ml complete culture medium to remove any residual Collagenase D solution.

9. Pellet the cells and resuspend in complete culture medium.

10. Count the cells and plate for immediate use (*see* **Note 10**).

4   Notes

1. A litter of 6–8 pups should yield approximately 20×10^6 to 25×10^6 cells. This protocol assumes all mice are of the same genotype and, therefore, all tissue digested together. If mice are of varying genotypes, tissue should be kept separate throughout the procedure and solution volumes scaled accordingly.

2. The addition of ascorbic acid to the culture medium is essential for chondrocyte maturation as it promotes the synthesis and secretion of collagen. β-glycerophosphate provides a phosphate source for proper mineralization of the maturing matrix [9, 10].

3. This procedure requires some practice. The dissection can either be performed in 1× PBS or on an absorbent bench pad moistened with 70 % ethanol. Care should be taken to avoid drying of the tissue during the procedure. When removing the viscera, care should be taken to not penetrate or open the bowel.

4. Decanting is preferred over aspiration as it is easy to lose tissue when aspirating. As mentioned in **Note 1**, if keeping tissue separate due to multiple genotypes, reduce the solution

volume appropriately. Conversely, increase the solution volume or use multiple conical tubes if digesting tissue from more than eight mice so that the tissue is freely floating. Constant agitation in the Pronase solution during this step will remove the majority of the soft tissue attached to the ribs and sterna.

5. This initial Collagenase D digestion results in the removal of any remaining soft tissue surrounding the ribs and sterna. It is not advisable to incubate the tissue in a shaking water bath at this point as this may begin to dissociate some of the chondrocytes that are desired in the final culture.

6. The cartilage tissues should appear clean of all soft tissue following this step. Be cautious when decanting as some of the ribs may begin to detach from the sterna by this point.

7. This second Collagenase D digestion is not only longer than the first, but uses a higher enzyme concentration. The goal of this digestion is to release the chondrocytes from their matrix. At the beginning of the incubation period, the tissue will appear as a tubular structure of cells, but by the end, the chondrocytes will be freely floating in the solution. The exact time of the incubation period will vary. Cell dissociation should be monitored under the microscope at least once per hour to avoid overdigestion. In addition to swirling the plate, dissociation can be encouraged by pipetting the tissue up and down several times.

8. Cells should be plated at high density for optimal results; 5×10^5 cells per well for 12-well plates and 1×10^6 cells per well for 6-well plates is recommended. 12-well plates work well for staining experiments (alkaline phosphatase and alizarin red). 6-well plates work well for mRNA and protein isolation. Cells should appear cuboidal with a granular cytoplasm once attached to the plate. If fibroblastic contaminating cells are abundant in the cultures, they can be removed by incubating with Trypsin for a few minutes without risking removal of the chondrocytes.

9. The femoral head cartilage from mice of the specified age (P21 to P28) will easily pinch off as a unit with blunt-ended forceps. This will not be the case in older mice. For older mice, the cartilage will need to be removed with a scalpel. Use of a dissection microscope may be helpful when shaving the cartilage with a scalpel as care should be taken to avoid isolation of the subchondral bone. The bone will appear opaque and brownish in color while the cartilage is translucent.

10. After plating, cells should appear cuboidal in shape. They will proliferate in culture, but dedifferentiate quickly and so should be used for experiments within 1 week following isolation.

References

1. Wu JJ, Weis MA, Kim LS et al (2010) Type III collagen, a fibril network modifier in articular cartilage. J Biol Chem 285:18537–18544

2. Han EH, Chen SS, Klisch SM et al (2011) Contribution of proteoglycan osmotic swelling pressure to the compressive properties of articular cartilage. Biophys J 101: 916–924

3. Zuscik MJ, Hilton MJ, Zhang X et al (2008) Regulation of chondrogenesis and chondrocyte differentiation by stress. J Clin Invest 118:429–438

4. Dao DY, Jonason JH, Zhang Y et al (2012) Cartilage-specific beta-catenin signaling regulates chondrocyte maturation, generation of ossification centers, and perichondrial bone formation during skeletal development. J Bone Miner Res 27:1680–1694

5. Kung MH, Yukata K, O'Keefe RJ et al (2012) Aryl hydrocarbon receptor-mediated impairment of chondrogenesis and fracture healing by cigarette smoke and benzo(a)pyrene. J Cell Physiol 227:1062–1070

6. Hanifi A, Richardson JB, Kuiper JH et al (2012) Clinical outcome of autologous chondrocyte implantation is correlated with infrared spectroscopic imaging-derived parameters. Osteoarthritis Cartilage 20:988–996

7. Halonen KS, Mononen ME, Jurvelin JS et al (2013) Importance of depth-wise distribution of collagen and proteoglycans in articular cartilage–a 3D finite element study of stresses and strains in human knee joint. J Biomech 46:1184–1192

8. Vaughan-Thomas A, Dudhia J, Bayliss MT et al (2008) Modification of the composition of articular cartilage collagen fibrils with increasing age. Connect Tissue Res 49:374–382

9. Gerstenfeld LC, Landis WJ (1991) Gene expression and extracellular matrix ultrastructure of a mineralizing chondrocyte cell culture system. J Cell Biol 112:501–513

10. Leboy PS, Vaias L, Uschmann B et al (1989) Ascorbic acid induces alkaline phosphatase, type X collagen, and calcium deposition in cultured chick chondrocytes. J Biol Chem 264: 17281–17286

Chapter 3

Isolating Endosteal Mesenchymal Progenitors from Rodent Long Bones

Ji Zhu, Valerie A. Siclari, and Ling Qin

Abstract

Bone marrow mesenchymal stem cells (MSCs) are promising therapeutic tools for tissue repair and the treatment of a number of human diseases. As a result, there is substantial interest in characterizing and expanding these cells to uncover their therapeutic potential. For preclinical studies, mesenchymal progenitors, containing both MSCs and their proliferative progeny, are commonly isolated from the central region of rodent long bones. However, challenges exist in expanding these central mesenchymal progenitors in culture. We have recently identified another population of progenitors within rodent long bones that resides close to the bone surface, which we termed endosteal mesenchymal progenitors. These cells are more metabolically active and more responsive to external stimuli compared to central mesenchymal progenitors and therefore, they represent a biologically important target for MSC research. This chapter describes in detail a unique enzymatic digestion approach to isolate and culture endosteal mesenchymal progenitors as well as their central counterparts from rodent long bones.

Key words Mesenchymal stem cells, Endosteal mesenchymal progenitors, Bone marrow, Enzymatic digestion, Colony forming unit-fibroblast

1 Introduction

Almost a half century ago, Alexander Friedenstein and colleagues pioneered a flushing method to isolate bone marrow cells from the central region of rodent long bones for culturing plastic-adherent and clonogenic fibroblastoid mesenchymal progenitors [1, 2]. Since then, the flushing method has become a standard technique to isolate mesenchymal progenitors from rodents in laboratories. Mesenchymal progenitor cultures are heterogeneous and consist of mesenchymal stem cells (MSCs), as well as their proliferative and more differentiated offspring [3]. In addition to their multilineage differentiation ability, these cells are immunosuppressive and capable of homing to injured tissues and secreting a number of bioactive molecules that promote wound repair and tissue regeneration. Therefore, they have been intensively investigated as

Jennifer J. Westendorf and Andre J. van Wijnen (eds.), *Osteoporosis and Osteoarthritis*, Methods in Molecular Biology, vol. 1226, DOI 10.1007/978-1-4939-1619-1_3, © Springer Science+Business Media New York 2015

potential therapeutic tools for tissue repair and for treatment of a number of diseases including Crohn's Disease and graft-versus-host disease [4]. However, these central mesenchymal progenitors are anatomically distant from trabecular and cortical bone surfaces where constant replenishment of bone forming osteoblasts by mesenchymal progenitors is required. There are also challenges associated with the rapid expansion of these cells in culture. For example, central mesenchymal progenitor cultures, especially those from mice, can be difficult to grow in vitro and have limited proliferative ability [5–8].

The endosteal bone marrow is the portion of the bone marrow that is close to the bone surface and in rodents, includes the bone marrow that is within the trabecular bone and close to the endocortical bone surface [9]. We have recently demonstrated that, in rodents, endosteal bone marrow cells contain a much higher frequency of mesenchymal progenitors than central bone marrow cells [8]. These endosteal mesenchymal progenitors have similar cell surface marker expression (rat: $CD90^+CD49e^+Nestin^+$ $CD45^-CD34^-$; mouse: $Sca-1^+CD105^+CD29^+CD73^+CD71^+CD44^+$ $CD45^-CD34^-$) and multilineage differentiation ability to central progenitors. However, they form much larger colony forming unit-fibroblast (CFU-F) colonies due to their higher proliferative ability and can be passaged more times in culture than their central counterparts. They also exhibit greater immunosuppressive activity both in vitro and in a mouse model of inflammatory bowel disease. Moreover, aging, a major contributing factor for osteoporosis, dramatically decreases their number, while injection of parathyroid hormone, an anabolic treatment for osteoporosis, strongly increases their number. We propose that these endosteal mesenchymal progenitors are a distinct population of progenitors that are more biologically relevant to skeletal homeostasis and disease than central mesenchymal progenitors [8]. In addition, endosteal mesenchymal progenitors may be more suitable for in vitro expansion for therapeutic treatment than central mesenchymal progenitors.

This chapter describes an enzymatic digestion method to isolate endosteal mesenchymal progenitors from rat and mouse long bones, along with the separate isolation of their central counterparts from the same bones. Methods to quantify, culture, and differentiate these cells are also described.

2 Materials

2.1 Animals

Sprague-Dawley rats or C57Bl/6 mice (*see* **Note 1**).

2.2 Instruments

1. Class II biological safety cabinet/cell culture hood and a horizontal laminar flow clean bench: both should be equipped with a UV light for decontamination.

2. Tissue culture incubator with temperature and gas composition controls.

3. Mini shaker that can be placed inside a tissue culture incubator.

4. Inverted microscope with phase-contrast ability.

5. Benchtop centrifuge with a swing-bucket rotor.

6. Sterile surgical scissors, surgical forceps, scalpel handles, and scalpel blades (#22).

7. Sterile 0.2 µm syringe filter.

8. Sterile 70 µm cell strainer.

9. Sterile 10 mL syringes with 25- and 27-G needles.

10. Sterile 15 and 50 mL polypropylene conical tubes.

11. Pipet-aid, sterile serological pipettes (5 and 10 mL) and gibson-type micropipettes and tips (20, 200, and 1,000 µL).

12. 25 cm^2 tissue culture flasks with vented seal caps, 100 mm tissue culture dishes, 100 mm petri dishes.

13. Hemocytometer.

2.3 Reagents and Media

1. 70 % ethanol.

2. Dulbecco's phosphate buffered saline (PBS).

3. Flushing medium: αMEM supplemented with 1 % fetal bovine serum (FBS), 100 IU/mL penicillin and 100 µg/mL streptomycin.

4. Protease solution: 2 mg/mL collagenase A (Roche Diagnostics, Indianapolis, IN) and 2.5 mg/mL trypsin dissolved in Dulbecco's PBS and filter sterilized using a syringe filter. This solution should be freshly prepared just before starting the isolation process.

5. Growth medium for rat mesenchymal progenitors: αMEM supplemented with 15 % FBS, 100 IU/mL penicillin, and 100 µg/mL streptomycin.

6. Growth medium for mouse mesenchymal progenitors: αMEM supplemented with 15 % FBS, 0.1 % β-mercaptoethanol, 20 mM glutamine, 100 IU/mL penicillin, and 100 µg/mL streptomycin.

7. Osteogenic medium: αMEM containing 10 % FBS, 10 nM dexamethasone, 10 mM β-glycerophosphate, and 50 µg/mL L-ascorbic acid (AA, *see* **Note 2**).

8. Adipogenic medium: αMEM with 10 % FBS, 0.5 mM isobuthylmethylxanthine, 10 mM indomethacin, 1 µM dexamethasone, and 10 µg/mL insulin.

9. Chondrogenic medium: DMEM with 10 % FBS, 0.1 µM dexamethasone, 50 µg/mL AA, 40 µg/mL L-proline, 100 µg/mL sodium pyruvate, 1 × ITS+, and 10 ng/mL TGFβ3.

10. 3 % acetic acid with methylene blue.

11. 3 % crystal violet in methanol.

12. 0.05 % trypsin/EDTA solution.

13. 0.4 % trypan blue solution.

3   Methods

3.1 Harvest of Rodent Hind Long Bones

1. Euthanize the animal by CO_2 inhalation.

2. Immediately transfer the dead animal to a clean bench prede-contaminated by UV radiation. Place the animal on a flat surface on its back and wet the pelt thoroughly with 70 % ethanol.

3. Using sterile forceps and scissors, incise and peel back the skin surrounding the hind long bones. Remove the bilateral hind long bones by cutting through the hip and ankle joints using sharp surgical scissors. Cut through the knee joint to separate the tibia and femur (*see* **Note 3**).

4. Place the long bones in a 100 mm petri dish filled with 10 mL of flushing medium. Transfer the petri dish with the bones to a tissue culture hood for bone marrow harvesting.

3.2 Isolation of Central and Endosteal Bone Marrow Cells

1. Under a sterile tissue culture hood, use forceps and a scalpel to remove all of the soft tissue surrounding the bones. After removal of the soft tissue, place the long bones into a new 100 mm petri dish filled with 10 mL of flushing medium.

2. Cut off both ends of the tibia and femur at the growth plate with a scalpel.

3. Fill a syringe with 5 (mouse) or 10 (rat) mL of flushing medium per animal (two tibiae and two femurs). Attach a 25- (rat) or 27-G needle (mouse) to the syringe and then place the filled syringe on the side of the work space.

4. Drill a hole at each end of the bones with a different needle and syringe.

5. With the prefilled syringe, place the needle in the hole at one end of the bone and press down the plunger to force medium through the bone. This will flush the bone marrow out of the bone through the opposite end of the bone.

6. Reverse the bone and repeat the flushing from the other end of the bone. Use 1 (mouse) or 2 (rat) mL of flushing medium to flush out each bone. Bone marrow cells released by flushing mainly come from the central part of the diaphyseal shaft and hence, are central bone marrow cells (Fig. 1, step 1, *see* **Note 4**). The bone marrow cells that are located in close proximity to the endosteum remain attached to the bone after the flushing

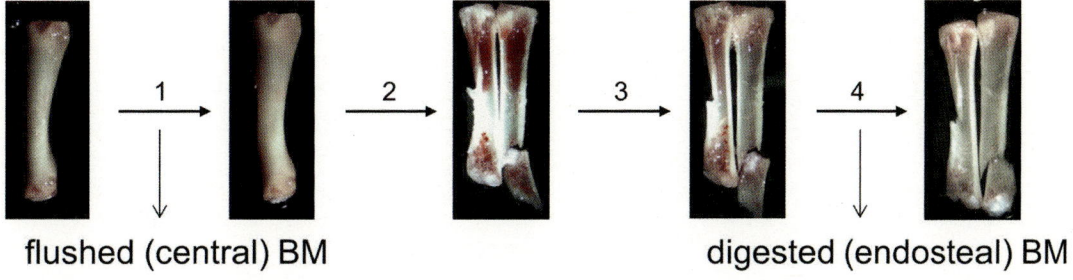

flushed (central) BM   digested (endosteal) BM

Fig. 1 Representative images of a rat femur during the isolation of endosteal bone marrow. *Step 1*: flush out central bone marrow cells from a bone that is free of its surrounding soft tissue and with both ends removed at the growth plates; *step 2*: predigest the whole bone to remove the periosteal progenitors and then longitudinally cut the bones into two halves; *step 3*: gently wash the bones to remove loosely attached bone marrow; *step 4*: digest bone fragments to collect endosteal bone marrow cells. BM: bone marrow. Reprinted from Bone, 53 (2), Siclari et al., Mesenchymal progenitors residing close to the bone surface are functionally distinct from those in the central bone marrow. 575–86, Copyright (2013), with permission from Elsevier

and are only released by enzymatic digestion (For information about how to culture central bone marrow mesenchymal progenitors, *see* **Note 5**).

7. After removing the central bone marrow cells, scrape the outside surface of the bones a few times with a scalpel blade and then place the bones into a 15 mL tube containing 5 mL of protease solution (eight mouse bones or four rat bones per tube).

8. Place the tubes on a mini shaker placed in the tissue culture incubator and shake for 20 min at 37 °C. This step removes periosteum and its associated periosteal progenitors from the long bones (Fig. 1 step 2, *see* **Note 6**).

9. After digestion, wash the bones with flushing medium, and then longitudinally cut the bones into two halves (Fig. 1 step 2, *see* **Note 7**).

10. Use a syringe to gently wash the inside of the bones with flushing medium to remove loosely attached bone marrow (Fig. 1 step 3, *see* **Note 8**).

11. Place the bone fragments into a 15 mL tube containing 5 mL of protease solution (eight mouse bones or four rat bones per tube) and perform the second digestion step for 60 min as described in **step 8** (Fig. 1 step 4).

12. Collect the supernatant and then add 5 mL of growth medium to neutralize the protease solution.

13. Centrifuge at $300 \times g$ for 5 min to pellet the cells.

14. Resuspend the cells in 5 mL of growth medium by gently pipetting up and down several times and then centrifuge.

15. Resuspend the cells in 3 mL of growth medium and then pass the cells through a cell strainer to remove debris (*see* **Note 9**).

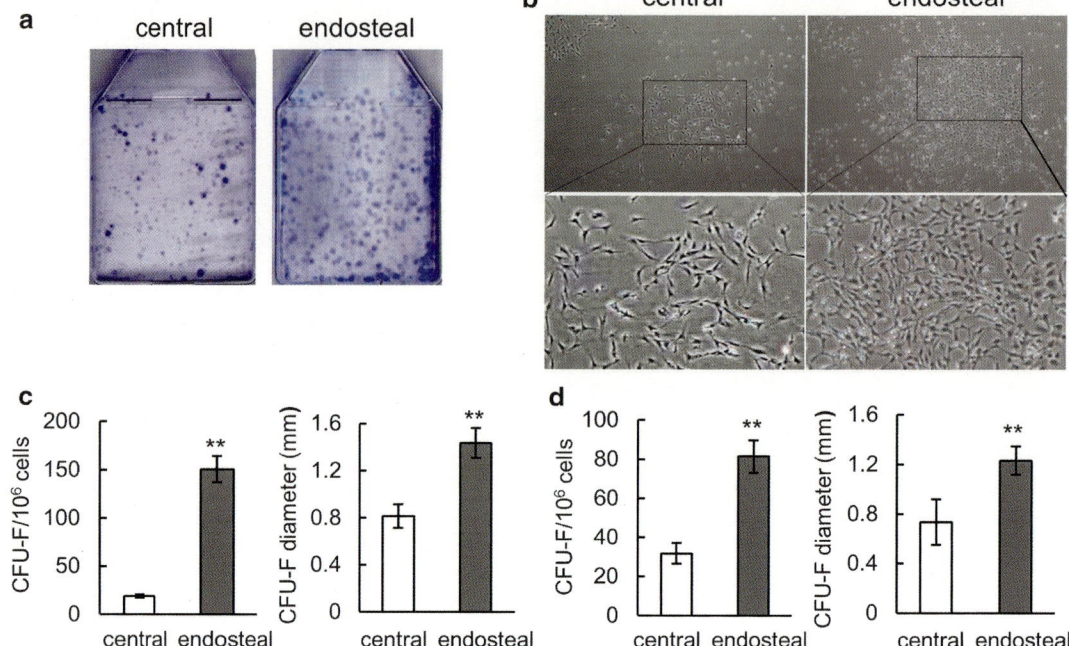

Fig. 2 CFU-F assays of rodent endosteal bone marrow cells compared to their central counterparts. (**a**) Representative images of 25 cm² flasks with mouse central and endosteal CFU-F colonies after staining. Note that the initial seeding densities are 3×10^6 and 1×10^6 cells per flask for central and endosteal bone marrow, respectively. (**b**) Representative images of mouse CFU-F colonies at low (*top*) and high (*bottom*) magnification. (**c**, **d**) Quantification of CFU-F frequency and diameter of endosteal bone marrow cells from mouse (**c**) and rat (**d**). **$p < 0.01$ vs. central

16. Perform a cell count by diluting a cell aliquot 1:10 in 3 % acetic acid with methylene blue to lyse the red blood cells.

17. Count the nucleated cells using a hemocytometer under a microscope. The expected cell recovery of endosteal bone marrow is $8–12 \times 10^6$ cells per mouse and $12–20 \times 10^6$ cells per rat.

3.3 CFU-F Assays of Endosteal Mesenchymal Progenitors

1. Seed 1×10^6 mononuclear endosteal bone marrow cells per 25 cm² flask in the growth medium and incubate the culture at 37 °C in 5 % CO_2 in a humidified tissue culture incubator (*see* **Note 10**).

2. Typically, after 5 (rat) or 7 (mouse) days of incubation, most colonies should contain more than 50 fibroblastic cells (Fig. 2a, b, *see* **Note 11**). At this point, remove medium and wash flasks twice with PBS.

3. Stain the colonies with 3 % crystal violet in methanol for at least 5 min.

4. Rinse flasks thoroughly with tap water to remove unbound stain.

5. Air-dry the flasks completely.

6. Count the number of CFU-F colonies under an inverted microscope with a 4× objective. We recommend drawing lines on the bottom of the flask to divide the surface into eight regions in order to facilitate counting. Only count colonies consisting of more than 50 cells. The expected CFU-F frequency of endosteal bone marrow cells is about 80–150 CFU-Fs per 1×10^6 mononuclear cells from both mouse and rat (Fig. 2c, d). The size of CFU-F colonies formed by endosteal bone marrow is normally larger than those formed by central bone marrow (Fig. 2c, d, *see* **Note 12**).

3.4 Culture and Differentiation of Endosteal Mesenchymal Progenitors

1. To culture endosteal mesenchymal progenitors, seed $3–5 \times 10^6$ mononuclear endosteal bone marrow cells per 100 mm tissue culture dishes in the growth medium and incubate at 37 °C in 5 % CO_2 in a humidified tissue culture incubator.

2. Change medium every 2–3 days.

3. When the cells reach 80–90 % confluence or when individual CFU-F colonies have expanded so that they are in close proximity to each other (about 8–10 days after plating), cells should be passaged for expansion. Aspirate the medium and wash the cells with PBS.

4. Add 3 mL of 0.05 % trypsin/EDTA to the cells and incubate for 2–3 min in the tissue culture incubator. Examine under the microscope to confirm that about 70–90 % of the cells are detached from the plate. If not, return the plate to the incubator for another 2 min. Typically, endosteal mesenchymal progenitors require less digestion time compared to central cells.

5. Neutralize the trypsin by adding 3 mL of growth medium and gently pipet up and down with a 10 mL serological pipette to obtain a single cell suspension.

6. Transfer the cells into a 15 mL tube and centrifuge at $300 \times g$ for 5 min at room temperature.

7. Resuspend the pellet in 3 mL of growth medium and count the number of cells. To count the number of live mesenchymal progenitors, dilute an aliquot of the cells in trypan blue solution to allow differentiation of live and dead cells. Count the number of live cells using a hemocytometer and a light microscope.

8. Plate the cells at a density of 0.5×10^6/100 mm dish. The cells that grow up are passage 1 cells.

9. Change medium every 2–3 days. Normally 80–90 % cell confluence is reached in 5–6 days. Lift and split cells at a ratio of 1:5 to 1:3 for expansion (*see* **Note 13**). The cells can also be stored in liquid nitrogen from passage 2–3 for future use.

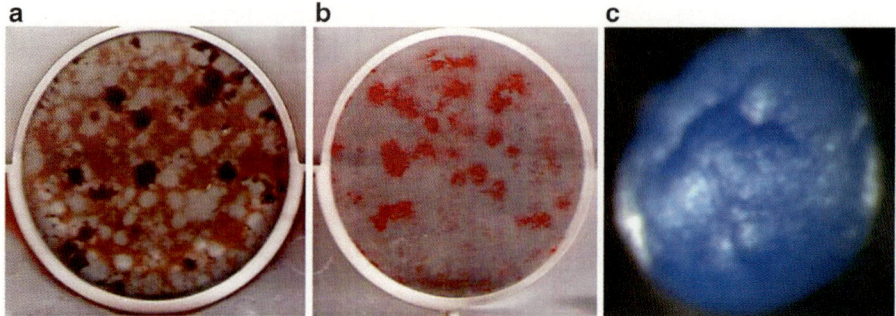

Fig. 3 Endosteal mesenchymal progenitors are capable of multilineage differentiation.(**a**) In vitro osteogenic differentiation as detected by von Kossa staining. (**b**) In vitro adipogenic differentiation as detected by oil red O staining. (**c**) In vitro micromass chondrogenic differentiation as detected by alcian blue staining

10. To differentiate the endosteal mesenchymal progenitors into osteoblast or adipocyte lineages (Fig. 3a, b), endosteal mesenchymal progenitors are first expanded to confluence in the growth medium and then switched to osteogenic or adipogenic medium, respectively, for 2–3 weeks. The differentiation media should be changed every 2–3 days.

11. To differentiate the endosteal mesenchymal progenitors into chondrocytes (Fig. 3c), seed a 20 μl droplet of 4×10^6 endosteal mesenchymal progenitors onto the center of a well in a 24-well plate. Two hours later, add 0.5 mL of chondrogenic medium. Change media every 3 days for about 3 weeks.

4   Notes

1. With this protocol, we have successfully isolated and cultured endosteal mesenchymal progenitors from 1 to 4-month-old Sprague-Dawley rats and 1 to 12-month-old C57Bl/6 mice. It is also compatible with other strains of mice we have tested, such as 129. The number of endosteal mesenchymal progenitors decreases significantly with aging [8]. Therefore, young animals (1–2-month-old) are the best source for obtaining these progenitors. In addition, the bones of young animals are much easier to cut while those from old animals tend to shatter and require more force during cutting (see **Note 7**).

2. Since ascorbic acid is very unstable and rapidly oxidizes in water, it should be freshly added to the medium from a frozen stock (50 mg/mL) just before changing medium on the cells.

3. Long bones should be harvested under sterile conditions. If a sterile clean bench is not available, long bones can be dissected in a tissue culture hood. Frequently dip the forceps and scissors in 70 % ethanol to prevent contamination into the cultures.

All procedures should be performed as quickly as possible to achieve a high yield of viable mesenchymal progenitors.

4. Be sure to hold the bone tightly with a pair of forceps during flushing to avoid dropping the bone. It is recommended to use a syringe with a screw-tip to prevent the needle from detaching from the syringe during flushing.

5. To culture central mesenchymal progenitors, flush the central bone marrow cells into a 50 mL conical tube. Gently pipet the cell suspension up and down to break up the clumps of bone marrow. Centrifuge the cells at $300 \times g$ for 5 min and resuspend the pellet in 5 mL of growth medium. Filter the cell suspension through a cell strainer and count the number of cells in the same way as described in **steps 16–17** of Subheading 3.2. The expected yield of central bone marrow is $30–50 \times 10^6$ cells per mouse and $120–200 \times 10^6$ cells per rat. Seed 3×10^6 cells per 25 cm² flask for CFU-F assays and $30–50 \times 10^6$ per 100 mm dish for expansion. CFU-F staining and counting are performed 7 (rat) and 10 (mouse) days later as described in Subheading 3.3. The expected frequency is about $20–50$ CFU-Fs$/1 \times 10^6$ mononuclear cells (Fig. 2c, d). Central mesenchymal progenitors are cultured in the same growth medium as endosteal mesenchymal progenitors but they grow much slower. Split central mesenchymal progenitors at a ratio of 1:2 or 1:3 when passaging.

6. It is important to remove all soft tissue, especially the periosteum, surrounding the long bones to avoid the contamination of mesenchymal progenitors from undesired sources. Periosteum contains periosteal progenitors that have similar characteristics to bone marrow mesenchymal progenitors [10]. Several previous studies also used collagenase digestion of flushed, minced, or chopped bone fragments to increase the yield of bone marrow mesenchymal progenitors [11–16]. However, they were likely to have contamination of periosteal progenitors because they did not remove the periosteum from the bone. We have demonstrated by histology that scraping and predigestion of the bones is sufficient to remove periosteal cells and therefore, prevent contamination of periosteal progenitors into the endosteal bone marrow [8].

7. Bones from old animals easily shatter during cutting. To minimize the amount of shattering, while holding the bone tightly with a pair of forceps, use a scalpel blade to first mark a longitudinal line on the outside of the bone surface. Then, slowly and forcefully cut along this line.

8. You can choose to harvest endosteal bone marrow cells from diaphyseal and metaphyseal regions separately. To do so, use a blade to cut the longitudinally halved bones at the junctions

between the metaphysis and diaphysis. Then, enzymatically digest the diaphyseal and metaphyseal bone fragments separately. We have found that the majority of endosteal mesenchymal progenitors reside in the metaphysis [8].

9. Endosteal bone marrow cells have a tendency to clump. If you intend to use these cells directly for flow cytometry, pass the cells through a cell strainer immediately before analyzing the cells by a flow cytometer.

10. We prefer using 25 cm^2 flasks over 6-well plates for CFU-F assays. Due to the concaved surface of the wells in a 6-well plate, we have found that the colonies tend to grow more at the center of the wells and become difficult to count individually. We have found the colonies to be more evenly distributed and easier to count in 25 cm^2 flasks.

11. Do not change the medium of cells plated for a CFU-F assay. Overall, minimize the amount of disturbance to the flasks after plating. If possible, allow the cells to remain undisturbed in the tissue culture incubator until it is time to count the cells. This ensures the optimal accuracy of the CFU-F assay.

12. The adherence and proliferative ability of mesenchymal progenitors varies significantly depending on culture conditions. It is recommended to test different batches of FBS in the growth medium to select one that gives the greatest number of CFU-Fs and optimal colony morphology and to use this one batch through the entire project.

13. To maintain a healthy cell population, it is advisable to passage cells at 80–90 % confluence and to avoid over-confluence. Endosteal mesenchymal progenitors grow much better and have a much shorter doubling time in culture than the commonly used central progenitors. While mouse central mesenchymal progenitors normally reach senescence and stop growth after 5–10 passages, we found that mouse endosteal mesenchymal progenitor cultures keep proliferating beyond 20 passages [8].

References

1. Friedenstein AJ, Chailakhjan RK, Lalykina KS (1970) The development of fibroblast colonies in monolayer cultures of guinea-pig bone marrow and spleen cells. Cell Tissue Kinet 3: 393–403

2. Friedenstein AJ, Gorskaja JF, Kulagina NN (1976) Fibroblast precursors in normal and irradiated mouse hematopoietic organs. Exp Hematol 4:267–274

3. Lindner U, Kramer J, Rohwedel J et al (2010) Mesenchymal stem or stromal cells: toward a better understanding of their biology? Transfus Med Hemother 37:75–83

4. Wang S, Qu X, Zhao RC (2012) Clinical applications of mesenchymal stem cells. J Hematol Oncol 5:19.5

5. Short B, Brouard N, Occhiodoro-Scott T et al (2003) Mesenchymal stem cells. Arch Med Res 34:565–571

6. Krishnappa V, Boregowda SV, Phinney DG (2013) The peculiar biology of mouse mesenchymal stromal cells–oxygen is the key. Cytotherapy 15:536–541

7. Banfi A, Muraglia A, Dozin B et al (2000) Proliferation kinetics and differentiation potential of ex vivo expanded human bone

marrow stromal cells: Implications for their use in cell therapy. Exp Hematol 28:707–715

8. Siclari VA, Zhu J, Akiyama K et al (2013) Mesenchymal progenitors residing close to the bone surface are functionally distinct from those in the central bone marrow. Bone 53:575–586

9. Ellis SL, Grassinger J, Jones A et al (2011) The relationship between bone, hemopoietic stem cells, and vasculature. Blood 118:1516–1524

10. van Gastel N, Torrekens S, Roberts SJ et al (2012) Engineering vascularized bone: osteogenic and proangiogenic potential of murine periosteal cells. Stem Cells 30:2460–2471

11. Morikawa S, Mabuchi Y, Kubota Y et al (2009) Prospective identification, isolation, and systemic transplantation of multipotent mesenchymal stem cells in murine bone marrow. J Exp Med 206:2483–2496

12. Xu S, De Becker A, Van Camp B et al (2010) An improved harvest and in vitro expansion protocol for murine bone marrow-derived mesenchymal stem cells. J Biomed Biotechnol 2010:105940

13. Nakamura Y, Arai F, Iwasaki H et al (2010) Isolation and characterization of endosteal niche cell populations that regulate hematopoietic stem cells. Blood 116:1422–1432

14. Ohishi M, Ono W, Ono N et al (2012) A novel population of cells expressing both hematopoietic and mesenchymal markers is present in the normal adult bone marrow and is augmented in a murine model of marrow fibrosis. Am J Pathol 180:811–818

15. Short BJ, Brouard N, Simmons PJ (2009) Prospective isolation of mesenchymal stem cells from mouse compact bone. Methods Mol Biol 482:259–268

16. Zhu H, Guo ZK, Jiang XX et al (2010) A protocol for isolation and culture of mesenchymal stem cells from mouse compact bone. Nat Protoc 5:550–560

Engineering Cartilage Tissue by Pellet Coculture of Chondrocytes and Mesenchymal Stromal Cells

Ling Wu, Janine N. Post, and Marcel Karperien

Abstract

Coculture of chondrocytes and mesenchymal stromal cells (MSCs) in pellets has been shown to be beneficial in engineering cartilage tissue in vitro. In these cultures trophic effects of MSCs increase the proliferation and matrix deposition of chondrocytes. Thus, large cartilage constructs can be made with a relatively small number of chondrocytes. In this chapter, we describe the methods for making coculture pellets of MSCs and chondrocytes. We also provide detailed protocols for analyzing coculture pellets with cell tracking, proliferation assays, species specific polymerase chain reactions (PCR), short tandem repeats analysis, and histological examination.

Key words Chondrocytes, Mesenchymal stromal cells, Coculture, Trophic effects, Cartilage engineering, Matrix deposition

1 Introduction

Partial replacement of chondrocytes by alternative cell sources can reduce the number of chondrocytes needed to engineering cartilage constructs in vitro [1–3]. Hendriks et al., cocultured bovine primary chondrocytes with human expanded chondrocytes, human dermal fibroblasts, mouse embryonic stem cells, mouse-3T3 feeder cells, or human mesenchymal stromal cells (MSCs) in cell pellets [4]. Their data indicated that cartilage matrix deposition increased in coculture pellets. Replacement of 80 % of the chondrocytes with other cell types resulted in similar amounts of GAG production when compared to pure chondrocyte pellets. This beneficial effect on cartilage formation is most prominent in cocultures of chondrocytes with mesenchymal stromal cells [5]. In a more recent study, we used a xenogeneic coculture model of human MSCs and bovine chondrocytes to study the contribution of each cell type to cartilage matrix formation [6, 7]. Our data showed a significant decrease in MSCs in coculture pellets over time, resulting in an almost homogeneous cartilage tissue predominantly derived from

Jennifer J. Westendorf and Andre J. van Wijnen (eds.), *Osteoporosis and Osteoarthritis*, Methods in Molecular Biology, vol. 1226, DOI 10.1007/978-1-4939-1619-1_4, © Springer Science+Business Media New York 2015

the initially seeded chondrocytes. Our data showed that the beneficial effect of coculture is largely due to increased chondrocyte proliferation and matrix formation, while chondrogenic differentiation of MSCs only marginally contributed to cartilage formation. We also demonstrated that these observations present in coculture pellets of chondrocytes and MSCs are independent of donor variation and culture conditions [8]. Subsequent experiments indicated that increased secretion of fibroblast growth factor 1 (FGF1) in coculture of MSCs and chondrocytes is responsible for increased chondrocyte proliferation in pellet cocultures [9]. Thrombospondin-2 has also been reported to be secreted by MSCs to promote chondrogenic differentiation both in vitro and in vivo [10]. These reports are the first to show the trophic role of MSCs in stimulating chondrocyte proliferation and matrix production.

2 Materials

2.1 Cell Sources

1. Bovine primary chondrocytes (bPCs) are isolated from full-thickness cartilage knee biopsies of female calves that are approximately 6 months old. Cartilage is separated and digested to extract primary chondrocytes (*see* Subheading 3.1).

2. Human primary chondrocytes (hPCs) are obtained from full thickness cartilage dissected from knee biopsies of a patient undergoing total knee replacement (*see* Subheading 3.2).

3. Human MSCs (hMSCs) are isolated from bone marrow aspirates of healthy donors (*see* **Note 1**).

2.2 Media, Solutions, Chemicals, and Kits

1. Chondrocyte proliferation medium: DMEM supplemented with 10 % FBS, 1 × nonessential amino acids, 0.2 mM ascorbic acid 2-phosphate (AsAP), 0.4 mM proline, 100 U penicillin/ml and 100 µg/ml streptomycin.

2. Chondrogenic differentiation medium: DMEM supplemented with 40 µg/ml of proline, 50 µg/ml ITS-premix, 50 µg/ml of AsAP, 100 µg/ml of Sodium Pyruvate, 10 ng/ml of Transforming Growth Factor beta 3 (TGFβ3), 10^{-7} M of dexamethasone, 500 ng/ml of Bone Morphogenetic Protein 6 (BMP6), 100 U penicillin/ml and 100 µg/ml streptomycin.

3. MSC proliferation medium:α-MEM plus 10 % fetal bovine serum, 1 % L-glutamine, 0.2 mM ascorbic acid, 100 U/ml penicillin, 10 µg/ml streptomycin and 1 ng/ml basic Fibroblast Growth Factor (bFGF).

4. Proteinase K digestion buffer: 1 mg/ml proteinase K (Sigma) in Tris–EDTA buffer (pH7.6), 18.5 µg/ml iodoacetamide and 1 µg/ml pepstatin A. The proteinase K solution can be stored

in aliquots at −20 °C for several weeks. After one thaw, do not freeze again. Tris–EDTA buffer: Dissolve 6.055 g Tris and 0.372 g EDTA · 2 H_2O in 1,000 ml of H_2O. Adjust pH to 7.6.

5. PBE buffer: 14.2 g/l Na_2HPO_4 and 3.72 g/l Na_2EDTA, pH 6.5.

6. GAG stock solution: 50 mg/ml, 17.5 mg of cysteine–HCl was dissolved in 10 ml of PBE buffer. Aliquoted and store in −20 °C freezer.

7. GAG working solution (200 μg/ml): Dilute GAG stock solution 1:250 in PBE buffer.

8. DMMB solution: add 9.5 ml of 0.1 M HCl solution to 90.5 ml of d_2H_2O plus 0.304 g of glycine and 0.237 g of NaCl; adjust to pH 3 before adding 1.6 mg of DMMB to the buffer. When stored in the dark at RT, the solution is stable for 3 months; filter to get rid of precipitates before use.

9. Organic fluorescent dye (CM-DiI), Click-iT® EdU Imaging Kit, and the CyQuant DNA Kit.

10. QIAamp DNA Mini Kit and RNeasy Mini Kit (Qiagen).

11. iScript cDNA Synthesis kit and iQ SYBR Green Supermix (Bio-Rad).

12. PowerPlex 16 System (Promega).

13. Collagenase type II (Worthington).

14. Click-iT® EdU Imaging Kit (Invitrogen).

15. Round bottom ultra low attachment 96-well plate.

16. Cryomatrix (Shandon).

17. DMMB (1, 9-Dimethyl-Methylene Blue).

2.3 Equipment

1. BD pathway 435 confocal microscope (BD Biosciences).

2. ELISA reader.

3. MyiQ2 Two-Color Real-Time PCR Detection System (Bio-Rad).

3 Methods

3.1 Isolation of Human Articular Chondrocytes

1. Human cartilage tissue were obtained from total knee or hip joint replacement.

2. Cartilage tissue is cut from underlying bone and connective tissue with scalpels and chopped into pieces of approximately 2 × 2 mm.

3. Digest cartilage pieces for 20–22 h in collagenase type II (0.15 %) in DMEM supplemented with penicillin (100 U/ml) and streptomycin (100 mg/ml).

3.2 Isolation of Human Bone Marrow Mesenchymal Stromal Cells

1. Collect bone marrow aspirates in sterile heparin tubes.

2. Pour aspirate into 50 ml Falcon tubes.

3. Remove red blood cells by incubating 100 µl aliquots of aspirate with 900 µl red blood cell lysing buffer for 5–10 min on ice or until transparent.

4. Count cell numbers with Trypan blue staining. Plate cells at 50,000/cm^2 in T75 in MSC proliferation medium plus 1 % heparin.

3.3 Cell Tracking of Cell Populations in Pellet Cocultures with Organic Fluorescent Dyes CM-DiI

1. Trypsinize bovine or human chondrocytes and resuspend in PBS at a concentration of 2×10^6 cells/ml.

2. Incubate the cells with the fluorescent dye CM-DiI (final concentration of 4 µM) at 37 °C for 5 min followed by incubation at 4 °C for 15 min.

3. Wash cells two times by suspending cells in PBS followed by collecting cells by centrifuging at $300 \times g$ for 3 min.

3.4 Coculture of bPCs and hMSCs in Pellets

1. Trypsinize hMSCs and suspend in chondrocyte proliferation medium at a concentration of 1×10^6 cells/ml. Resuspend labeled bPCs or hPCs from Subheading 3.1 at the same concentration as hMSCs in chondrocyte proliferation medium.

2. Mix hMSCs with bPCs or hPCs at ratios of 80/20 % and 50/50 %. Seed a total of 200,000 cells in one well of a round bottom ultra low attachment 96-well plate in chondrocyte proliferation medium.

3. Use mono-culture of hMSCs only or bPCs only or hPCs only as controls. Cell numbers per well are the same as in coculture pellets.

4. Make pellets by centrifugation of the plate at $500 \times g$ for 5 min.

5. Xenogeneic cocultures (bPCs and hMSCs), including corresponding controls, are cultured in chondrocyte proliferation medium at all times.

6. For allogenic cocultures (hPCs and hMSCs), including corresponding controls, medium is changed to chondrogenic differentiation medium (*see* Subheading 2.2) on the second day after seeding.

3.5 Examination of Cell Proliferation in Pellets by EdU Labeling and Staining

1. 2 or 3 days after making pellets, add EdU (5-ethynyl-2′-deoxyuridine, provided in Click-iT® EdU Imaging Kit) to the culture medium of pellets at a concentration of 10 µM.

2. Harvest samples for analysis, 24 h later by transferring pellets to eppendorf tubes.

3. Wash cell pellets with PBS and fix with 10 % formalin for 15 min.

4. Embed samples in cryomatrix, and cut 10 μM sections with a cryotome.

5. Permeabilize sections and stain for EdU with Click-iT® EdU Imaging Kit according to the manufacturer's protocol. In this kit, nuclei are counterstained with LP435 (Hoechst 33342, provided in Click-iT® EdU Imaging Kit).

3.6 Image Acquisition and Analysis by Fluorescent Microscopy

1. Make fluorescent images with a BD pathway 435 confocal microscope (*see* **Note 2**).

2. Capture three separate images for each pellet section, using BP536/40 (Alexa 488), BP593/40 (DiI), and LP435 (Hoechst 33342) and pseudo color green, red, and blue respectively.

3. Open blue image of one pellet section with ImageJ software [11].

4. Set threshold by click drop-down menu via Image→ Adjust→Threshold (*see* **Note 3**).

5. Open particle analyzer via Analyze→analyze particles.

6. Set area restrictions: 100-infinite; choose Display results, Exclude on edges, Include holes; click OK to count NUMBER $_{\text{of total cell}}$ (*see* **Note 4**).

7. Open red image of the same pellet section; set threshold as described above (*see* **Note 5**).

8. Open image calculator via Process→Image calculator.

9. Select blue image in the box of Image 1; select red image in the box of Image 2; select "AND" in the box of Operation; then click OK to generate a new image named "result of blue."

10. Run "Analyze particles" on new image "result of blue" with the same setting as above to count NUMBER $_{\text{of red cell}}$.

11. Open green image of the same pellet; set threshold and area restriction (*see* **step 6**) to count NUMBER $_{\text{of green cell}}$.

12. Run "Image calculator" by selecting green image in Image 1 box and red image in Image 2 box, with AND in Operation box to generate new image named "result of green."

13. Run "Analyze particles" on new image "result of green" with same setting as above to count NUMBER $_{\text{of green plus red cell}}$.

14. Input all NUMBERs into an Excel spreadsheet and perform the following calculations: Rate of EdU positive Chondrocyte = NUMBER $_{\text{of green plus red cell}}$ ÷ NUMBER $_{\text{of red cell}}$ × 100 %; Rate of EdU positive MSCs = (NUMBER $_{\text{of green cell}}$ − NUMBER $_{\text{of green plus red cell}}$) ÷ (NUMBER $_{\text{of total cell}}$ − NUMBER $_{\text{of red cell}}$) × 100 %; Labeling efficiency = NUMBER $_{\text{of red cell}}$ ÷ NUMBER $_{\text{of total cell}}$ × 100 % (*see* **Note 6**).

Table 1
Series dilution of GAG standards

GAG amount	Blank	0.5 µg	1 µg	1.5 µg	2 µg	2.5 µg
GAG working solution (*see* **Note 9**)	0 µl	10 µl	20 µl	30 µl	40 µl	50 µl
PBE buffer (*see* **Note 10**)	100 µl	90 µl	80 µl	70 µl	60 µl	50 µl

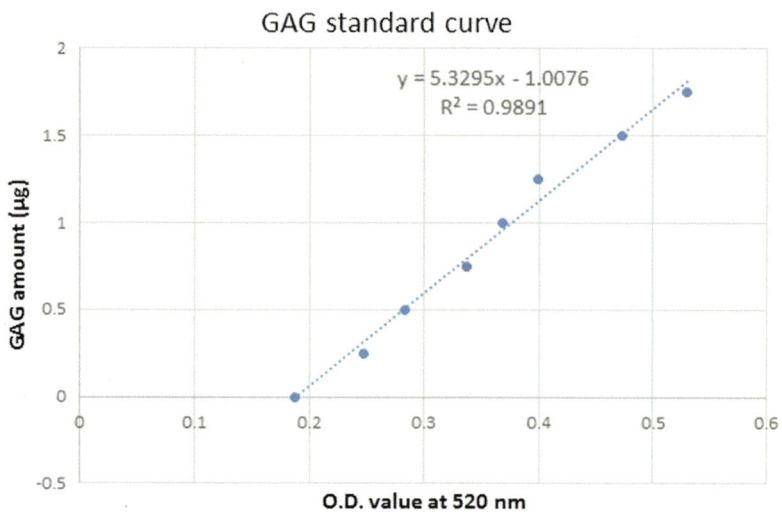

Fig. 1 An example of standard curve for GAG quantification. The blank (25 µl PBE, 5 µl 2.3 M NaCl and 150 µl DMMB solution) has an O.D. value of 0.18 ± 0.03

3.7 Quantitative GAG and DNA Assay

1. Perform glycosaminoglycan (GAG) and DNA assay at the end of coculture (i.e. 4 weeks).

2. Wash cell pellets ($n=6$) with PBS and freeze pellets overnight at −80 °C.

3. Digest pellets in 500 µl of proteinase K digestion buffer (*see* **Note 7**) for more than 16 h at 56 °C.

4. To prepare a standard curve, make dilution series of cysteine–HCl, according to Table 1.

5. Add 5 µl of a 2.3 M NaCl solution and 25 µl of the samples or the standard in one well of a 96-well nontissue-culture-treated plate.

6. Add 150 µl of the DMMB (1, 9-Dimethyl-Methylene Blue) solution (*see* Subheading 2.2) and read the absorbance at 520 nm on an ELISA reader. Figure 1 gives an example of a standard curve (*see* Subheading 2.2).

7. Determine cell number by quantification of total DNA using a CyQuant DNA Kit, according to the manufacturer's instructions.

3.8 Cell Tracking with Species Specific PCR

1. Perform species-specific PCR to determine the ratio of MSCs and chondrocytes in xenogeneic coculture (hMSCs and bPCs) pellets at the end of culture (i.e. 4 weeks).

2. Isolate DNA samples of pellets with a QIAamp DNA Mini Kit according to the manufacturer's protocols.

3. Extract RNA samples of pellets with an RNeasy Mini Kit (*see* **Note 8**).

4. Reverse-transcribe one microgram of total RNA into cDNA using the iScript cDNA Synthesis kit.

5. Perform species-specific quantitative PCR (qPCR) on genomic DNA or cDNA samples by using the iQ SYBR Green Supermix.

6. Carry out PCR Reactions on MyiQ2 Two-Color Real-Time PCR Detection System under the following conditions: Denature cDNA for 5 min at 95 °C, follow with 45 cycles consisting of 15 s at 95 °C, 15 s at 60 °C and 30 s at 72 °C.

7. Generate a melting curve for each reaction to test primer dimer formation and nonspecific priming.

8. The primers for real-time PCR, either species specific or cross species-specific, are listed in Tables 2 and 3.

9. For each gene, standard curves are obtained by serial dilutions of cDNA (*see* **Note 9**). Figure 2 gives an example of standard curve for qPCR.

10. Use Bio-Rad iQ5 optical system software (version 2.0) to calculate copy numbers for each condition using the standard curve as reference.

11. Ratio of bovine or human cells in the xenogenic coculture pellets are defined as the proportion of human or bovine GAPDH copy numbers as percentage of the total copy numbers

Table 2
Forward (F) and reverse (R) primers used for quantitative PCR on genomic DNA

Gene name	Primer sequence	Product size	Gene bank No.
Cross-species GAPDH	F: 5′ GCATTGCCCTCAACGACCA 3′ R: 5′ CACCACCCTGTTGCTGTAGCC 3′	179 or 171[a]	NC_000012 and NC_007303
Human-specific GAPDH	F: 5′ TTCCACCCATGGCAAATTCC 3′ R: 5′ TTGCCTCCCCAAAGCACATT 3′	131	NC_000012
Bovine-specific GAPDH	F: 5′ AGCCGCATCCCTGAGACAAG 3′ R: 5′ CAGAGACCCGCTAGCGCAAT 3′	132	NC_007303

[a]Product size of human genomic GAPDH is 179, of bovine genomic GAPDH is 171

Table 3
Forward (F) and reverse (R) primers used for quantitative RT-PCR

Gene name	Primer sequence	Product size	Gene bank No.
Cross-species β-Actin	F: 5′ GCGCAAGTACTCCGTGTGGA 3′ R: 5′ AAGCATTTGCGGTGGACGAT 3′	123	NM_001101 and NM_173979
Cross-species GAPDH	F: 5′ AGCTCACTGGCATGGCCTTC 3′ R: 5′ CGCCTGCTTCACCACCTTCT 3′	116	NM_002046 and NM_001034034
Human-specific GAPDH	F: 5′ CGCTCTCTGCTCCTCCTGTT 3′ R: 5′CCATGGTGTCTGAGCGATGT 3′	82	NM_002046
Bovine-specific GAPDH	F: 5′ GCCAT CACTG CCACC CAGAA 3′ R: 5′ GCGGCAGGTCAGATCCACAA 3′	207	NM_001034034
Human-specific aggrecan	F: 5′ TTCCCATCGTGCCTTTCCA 3′ R: 5′ AACCAACGATTGCACTGCTCTT 3′	121	NM_013227
Bovine-specific aggrecan	F: 5′ CCAAGCTCTGGGGAGGTGTC 3′ R: 5′ GAGGGCTGCCCACTGAAGTC 3′	98	NM_173981
Human-specific collagen II	F: 5′ GGCGGGGAGAAGACGCAGAG 3′ R: 5′ CGCAGCGAAACGGCAGGA 3′	129	NM_001844
Bovine-specific collagen II	F: 5′ AGGTCTGACTGGCCCCATTG 3′ R: 5′ CTCGAGCACCAGCAGTTCCA 3′	101	NM_001001135
Human-specific collagen IX	F: 5′ GGCAGAAATGGCCGAGACG 3′ R: 5′ CCCTTTGTTAAATGCTCGCTGA 3′	150	NM_001851
Bovine-specific collagen IX	F: 5′GGACTCAACACGGGTCCACA 3′ R: 5′ ACAGGTCCAGCAGGGCTTTG 3′	102	XM_601325

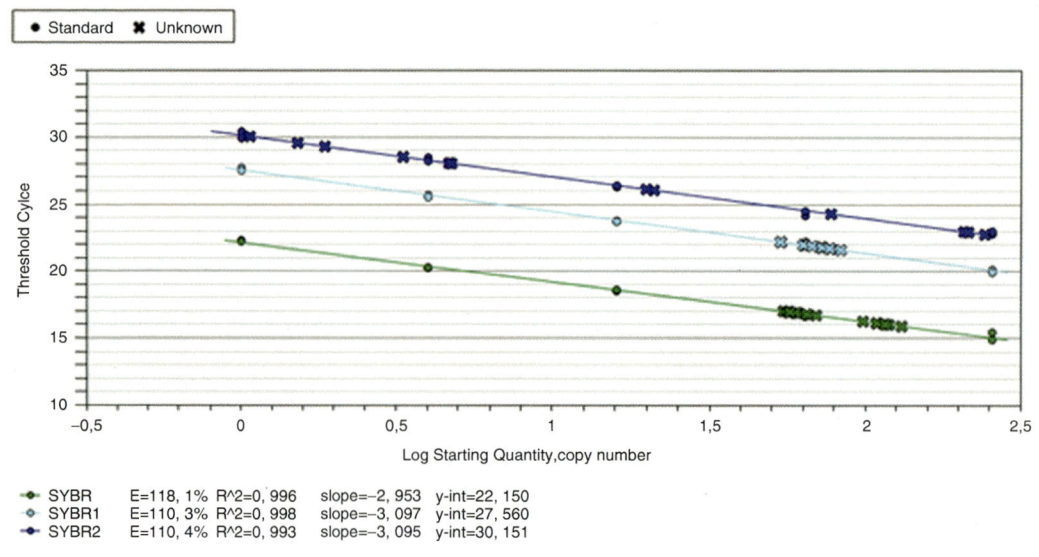

SYBR   E=118, 1% R^2=0, 996   slope=−2, 953   y-int=22, 150
SYBR1   E=110, 3% R^2=0, 998   slope=−3, 097   y-int=27, 560
SYBR2   E=110, 4% R^2=0, 993   slope=−3, 095   y-int=30, 151

Fig. 2 An example of standard curve for qPCR. SYBR, SYBR1, and SYBR2 stand for three different primer sets

of both human and bovine genes determined by species specific PCR using genomic DNA as a template.

12. The relative mRNA expression level of bovine or human genes in xenogenic cocultures is determined by normalizing the values using cross species-specific GAPDH and β-actin primers.

3.9 Short Tandem Repeats (STR) Analysis

1. Perform STR analysis to determine the ratio of MSCs and chondrocytes in allogeneic cocultures (hMSCs and hPCs) pellets.

2. Extract genomic DNA samples from pellets ($n=6$) with the QIAamp DNA Mini Kit.

3. Amplify the 16 loci of the kit PowerPlex 16 System, type "sequence," and analyze all loci according to manufacturer's protocol.

4. Compare mono-cultures of hMSCs or hPCs to find informative alleles only present in either the hMSCs or the hPCs donor (*see* **Note 10**).

5. Make electropherograms of the informative loci.

6. As shown in Fig. 3, calculate the area under the peaks, which stand for the abundancy of the alleles.

7. The sum of the area under the peak for the two donor specific alleles represents a relative amount of DNA for this donor.

8. Calculate the relative DNA amount for both the hMSC and the hPC donor.

9. Calculate the ratio of hMSCs and hPCs in the pellet by dividing through the total amount of relative DNA present in the pellet.

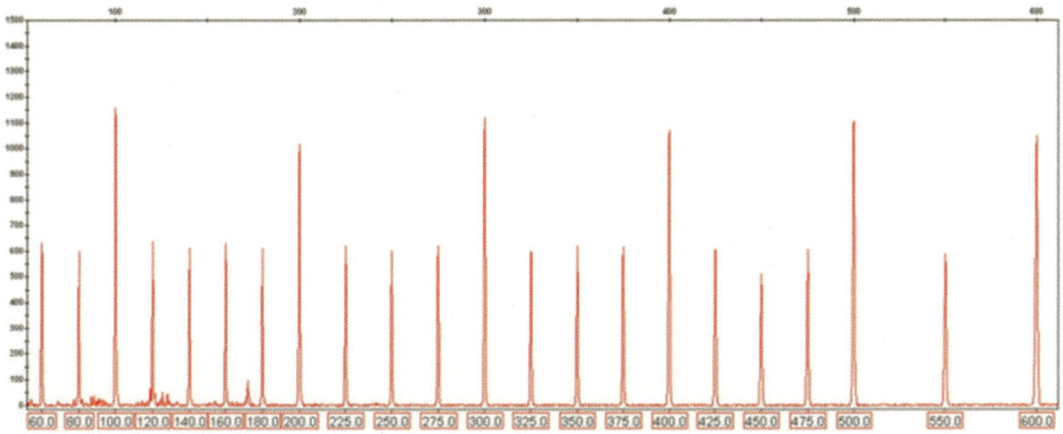

Fig. 3 An example of electropherogram of fragments after amplification. Adapted from the instructions of use of the "PowerPlex® 16 System" provided by Promega. Copyright to Promega

4 Notes

1. We define the "primary" cells (bPCs, hPCs, and hMSCs) in this manuscript as cells with low passage number (<2) without immortalization.

2. Using montage capture, images of high resolutions were obtained covering the entire section of a pellet. Choose the 20× objective. Use standard setting for the microscope and software.

3. Thresholds can usually be set by clicking "Dark background" option on the "Threshold window". If large artifacts appear, set threshold manually by adjusting the threshold bars so that the objects are red; click set and then ok.

4. By setting 100-infinite, any artifacts smaller than 100 pixel^2 (10×10 pixel) will be excluded. In images made with 20× objective, cell nuclei (either bovine or human) are larger than 100 pixel^2.

5. Setting the threshold for red image is tricky. Labeling efficiency is calculated to estimate the accuracy of threshold setting. Labeling efficiency should be similar to the ratio of chondrocytes used to establish the cocultures particularly in early time points (up to a few days maximum) after establishing the culture.

6. It is possible to automatically analyze all images by running customized plugins, which are written specifically for counting cells in different colors, using macro language of ImageJ. Basic knowledge about computer programing is required. Our plugin is available upon request.

7. Reading of absorbance at 520 nm gives variations. Always do triplicates for standards and samples.

8. Coculture pellets usually contain a lot of extracellular matrix, which makes it very difficult to extract RNA. After washing with PBS, pellets must be snap frozen with liquid nitrogen and smashed with pestle and mortar. Add lysis buffer to mortar to collet total RNA. To get 1 μg of RNA, at least three pellets (200,000 cells per pellet) are needed.

9. Take equal amount of cDNA from all samples in the same experiment to make a stock solution of cDNA templates. From the stock solution, make a series dilution: 1×, 4×, 16×, 64×, and 256× times. Run standards on the same plate as Unknown (samples to be tested), then make standards curves with Ct values in Bio-Rad iQ5 optical system software (version 2.0).

10. Theoretically, a random pair of human individuals has at least one locus (within the 16 loci tested in the kit), which is informative, except for identical twins. Normally, 2-3 loci are informative to distinguish the hMSC and the hPC donor at the DNA level.

References

1. Wu L, Cai X, Zhang S et al (2013) Regeneration of articular cartilage by adipose tissue derived mesenchymal stem cells: perspectives from stem cell biology and molecular medicine. J Cell Physiol 228:938–944

2. Leijten JCH, Georgi N, Wu L et al (2013) Cell sources for articular cartilage repair strategies: shifting from monocultures to cocultures. Tissue Eng Part B Rev 19:31–40

3. Moreira-Teixeira LS, Georgi N, Leijten J et al (2011) Cartilage tissue engineering. Endocr Dev 21:102–115

4. Hendriks JAA, Miclea RL, Schotel R et al (2010) Primary chondrocytes enhance cartilage tissue formation upon co-culture with a range of cell types. Soft Matter 6: 5080–5088

5. Acharya C, Adesida A, Zajac P et al (2012) Enhanced chondrocyte proliferation and mesenchymal stromal cells chondrogenesis in coculture pellets mediate improved cartilage formation. J Cell Physiol 227:88–97

6. Wu L, Leijten JC, Georgi N et al (2011) Trophic effects of mesenchymal stem cells increase chondrocyte proliferation and matrix formation. Tissue Eng Part A 17:1425–1436

7. Hildner F, Concaro S, Peterbauer A et al (2009) Human adipose-derived stem cells contribute to chondrogenesis in coculture with human articular chondrocytes. Tissue Eng Part A 15:3961–3969

8. Wu L, Prins HJ, Helder MN et al (2012) Trophic effects of mesenchymal stem cells in chondrocyte co-cultures are independent of culture conditions and cell sources. Tissue Eng Part A 18:1542–1551

9. Wu LG, Leijten J, van Blitterswijk C et al (2013) Fibroblast growth factor -1 is a mesenchymal stromal cell secreted factor stimulating proliferation of osteoarthritic chondrocytes in co-culture. Stem Cells Dev 22: 2356–2367

10. Jeong SY, Kim DH, Ha J et al (2013) Thrombospondin-2 secreted by human umbilical cord blood-derived mesenchymal stem cells promotes chondrogenic differentiation. Stem Cells 31:2136–2148

11. Abramoff MD, Magalhaes PJ, Ram SJ (2004) Image processing with ImageJ. Biophoton Int 11:36–42

Chapter 5

Generation of Induced Pluripotent Stem Cells

David R. Deyle

Abstract

Induced pluripotent stem cells (iPSCs) are generated from somatic cells that have been reprogrammed by the ectopic expression of defined embryonic transcription factors. This technology has provided investigators with a powerful tool for modelling disease and developing treatments for human disorders. This chapter provides the researcher with some background on iPSCs and details on how to produce MEF-conditioned medium, prepare mitotically arrested mouse embryonic fibroblasts (MEFs), create iPSCs using viral vectors, passage iPSCs, and cryopreserve iPSCs. The methods offered here have been used in many laboratories around the world and the reader can initially follow these methods. However, not all cell types are easily transduced using viral vectors and other methods of delivering the reprogramming transcription factors may need to be tested.

Key words Induced pluripotent stem cells, Pluripotency, Reprogramming, iPSC isolation, Mouse embryonic fibroblasts, Cryopreservation, iPSC passaging

1 Introduction

In 2006, a major advance in stem cell biology was reported by Takahashi and Yamanaka [1]. They showed that after the introduction of a combination of different transcription factors by retroviral transduction into mouse embryonic fibroblasts could be reprogrammed into embryonic-like cells, designated induced pluripotent stem cells. Within the next year, Takahashi et al. [2] and Yu et al. [3] had adapted this technology for the successful reprogramming of human somatic cells (skin fibroblasts). To be reprogrammed, somatic cells must ectopically express four transcription factors *OCT4*, *SOX2*, *KLF4* or *MYC*, and *NANOG* or *LIN28*. Fully reprogrammed human iPSCs express the embryonic antigens SSEA3, TRA-1-60, TRA-1-81, DNMT3β, and REX1 [4] and have the capacity to differentiate into the three germ layers, mesoderm, ectoderm, and endoderm. Like embryonic stem cells, human iPSCs can divide infinitely and be differentiated into all somatic cell types.

Jennifer J. Westendorf and Andre J. van Wijnen (eds.), *Osteoporosis and Osteoarthritis*, Methods in Molecular Biology, vol. 1226, DOI 10.1007/978-1-4939-1619-1_5, © Springer Science+Business Media New York 2015

Since the first iPSC experiment, many alternative methods of generating iPSCs have been developed, including ones that use integrating, excisable, and non-integrating viral vectors, as well as non-viral systems. Each of these methods has its own advantages and disadvantages, which are discussed in a review by Robinton and Daley [5]. Fibroblasts have been the most common cell type to reprogram, likely because these cells are readily available or can be safely obtained by skin biopsy and are easy to culture in the laboratory. A number of different cell types, such as neural stem cells, liver cells, keratinocytes, amniotic cells, adipose cells, bone marrow stromal cells, and blood cells, have also been reprogrammed into iPSCs using a variety of different reprogramming methods. This chapter describes a method of generating iPSC from fibroblasts or mesenchymal stem cells using two different forms of integrating viruses.

2   Materials

2.1   Reagents

1. Dispase.

2. Phosphate-buffered saline (PBS), without Ca++ or Mg++, pH 7.4.

3. Dulbecco's modified Eagle's media/nutrient mixture F-12 (DMEM/F12) with GlutaMAX and sodium pyruvate.

4. Knockout Serum Replacement (Knockout SR) (Invitrogen).

5. Penicillin/streptomycin (Pen/Strep).

6. Nonessential amino acids (NEAA).

7. β-Mercaptoethanol.

8. Recombinant human fibroblast growth factor basic (bFGF).

9. DMEM high glucose (Cellgro).

10. Heat-inactivated fetal bovine serum (FBS).

11. Trypsin.

12. Dimethyl sulfoxide.

13. Gelatin.

14. Rho-associated protein kinase (ROCK) inhibitor (Millipore) (*see* **Note 1**).

15. Defined, serum-free cryopreservation medium (mFreSR) (Stem Cell Technologies).

16. Trypan blue, 0.4 %.

17. Lentiviral (LV) reprogramming vectors for transduction (*see* **Note 2**).

(a) LV-OCT4.

(b) LV-SOX2.

    (c) LV-LIN28.

    (d) LV-NANOG.

18. Polybrene.

19. Foamy viral reprogramming vector (ΔΦ53MOSKMETNW) (*see* **Note 3**).

20. Passage 2 (P2), DR4 mouse embryonic fibroblasts (MEFs) (*see* **Note 4**).

21. DMEM low glucose.

22. L-Glutamine.

2.2 Equipment

1. Laminar flow biological safety cabinet.

2. Incubator, water jacketed and humidified with 5 % CO_2, maintained at 37 °C.

3. Centrifuge with swinging bucket rotor, capable of holding various tube sizes.

4. Inverted microscope with interference phase optics.

5. Dissecting microscope.

6. Glass hemocytometer.

7. Vacuum aspiration source with tubing and waste container.

8. 37 °C water bath.

9. Electric or manual pipette filler/dispenser.

10. −80 °C freezer.

11. Liquid nitrogen dewar storage unit.

12. Bunsen burner.

13. P20, P200, P1000 pipettes.

14. Irradiator.

15. Isopropanol freezing containers.

2.3 Special Equipment/Supplies for Freezing iPSCs in Straws

1. Bio-Cool III controlled-rate freezer.

2. Sterile plugged Cassou straws (Veterinary Concepts, #04170).

3. Plastic goblet cylindrical holder for loaded straws (Veterinary Concepts, #04910).

4. Aluminum cryocanes.

5. Methanol.

6. Very long forceps.

2.4 Supplies

1. Cotton plugged, sterile Pasteur pipettes 5 ¾ in. and a bulb.

2. 5, 10, and 25 ml sterile serological pipettes.

3. 50 ml sterile conical centrifuge tubes.

4. 15 ml sterile conical centrifuge tubes.

5. P20, P200, P1000 filtered, sterilized tips.

6. Nunc cell culture cryogenic tubes (cryovials).

7. 6-, 12-, and 24-well tissue culture plates.

8. 35, 60, and 100 mm tissue culture dishes.

9. Sterile 100, 250, 1,000 ml bottles.

10. 1 ml syringe.

11. Straw Adapter, 1/4 cc (Veterinary Concepts).

2.5 Working Solutions

1. bFGF solution: 10 μg bFGF (*see* **Note 5**), 1 ml PBS, and 20 μl Knockout SR. Dispense into 8–125 μl aliquots and store FGF solution at –20 °C.

2. Human embryonic stem cell medium (HESCM): 500 ml DMEM/F12 with GlutaMAX and sodium pyruvate, 100 ml Knockout SR (final conc. ~17 %), 6 ml Pen/Strep (final conc. ~1 %), 6 ml NEAA (final conc. ~1 %), bFGF (final conc. 2 ng/ml) (*see* **Note 5**), 0.6 ml 0.1 M β-mercaptoethanol (0.35 ml β-mercaptoethanol in 50 ml H_2O). Pass medium through 0.22 μm filter into sterile bottle. The medium can be stored at 4 °C for 14 days. Before an experiment, warm the medium to 37 °C.

3. Dispase: 100 ml PBS, 100 mg of dispase (final conc. 1 mg/ml). Pass dispase through 0.22 μm filter into sterile bottle. Dispase can be stored at 4 °C for 7 days. Before an experiment, warm dispase to room temperature.

4. MEF culture medium: 500 ml DMEM high glucose, 50 ml FBS (final conc. ~10 %), and 5 ml Pen/Strep (final conc. ~1 %). The medium can be stored at 4 °C for 14 days. Before an experiment, warm the medium to 37 °C.

5. Mesenchymal stem cell medium (MSCM): 500 ml DMEM low glucose, 50 ml FBS (final conc. ~10 %), 5 ml L-glutamine, and 5 ml Pen/Strep (final conc. ~1 %). The medium can be stored at 4 °C for 14 days. Before an experiment, warm the medium to 37 °C.

6. Gelatin stock: 100 g of gelatin in 1000 ml of double-distilled water and autoclave. 0.5 % gelatin stock solution can be stored at room temperature.

7. Gelatin working solution: 100 ml of 0.5 % gelatin stock solution plus 400 ml sterile water. 0.1 % gelatin working solution can be stored at room temperature.

8. MEF freeze medium (FM): 50 % MEF culture medium, 40 % FBS, and 10 % DMSO.

9. Straw freezing medium (FMs): 70 % HESCM, 20 % knockout SR, and 10 % DMSO.

10. Cryovial freezing medium (FMc): mFreSR plus 10 μM ROCK inhibitor.

3 Methods

3.1 Expansion of Passage 2 DR4 MEFs

This protocol is based on Xu et al. [6]. We use passage 3 (P3) MEFs for the production of MEF-conditioned medium. It is best to expand P2 DR4 MEFs (*see* **Note 6**) and freeze cells for later use.

1. Thaw vial of P2 DR4 MEFs by placing vial of cells in 37 °C water bath without submersing the cap. Swirl gently.

2. When no crystals remain, wipe vial with 70 % ethanol and place in cell culture hood.

3. Use a sterile pipette to transfer cells to 50 ml conical tube containing 5 ml MEF culture medium.

4. Centrifuge at $800 \times g$ for 5 min.

5. Aspirate medium and resuspend cells in 10 ml of MEF culture medium.

6. Add 1 ml of cell suspension to 100 mm dish for a total of ten dishes.

7. Add 9 ml of MEF culture medium and gently rock dish to disperse cells evenly.

8. Place cells in 37 °C incubator.

9. Aspirate medium and add 10 ml new MEF culture medium every 3 days.

10. When cells are confluent, aspirate medium and wash cells with 4 ml PBS.

11. Add 2 ml 0.05 % trypsin to each dish and incubate at 37 °C for 3–5 min.

12. Collect using MEF culture medium and pool into a 50 ml conical tube.

13. Centrifuge at $800 \times g$ for 5 min.

14. As cells are spinning, make fresh FM.

15. Aspirate medium off cells and resuspend cells in 10 ml of FM.

16. Place 1 ml of cell suspension in cryovial, put in room-temperature isopropanol freezing containers, and place containers in –80 °C overnight.

17. The next day store cryogenic tubes in liquid nitrogen. Alternately, MEF-conditioned medium can be produced immediately following the expansion of MEFs.

18. When cells are confluent, aspirate medium and wash 8 dishes with 4 ml PBS. Save remaining dishes for generation of MEF-conditioned medium.

19. Add 2 ml 0.05 % trypsin to each dish and incubate at 37 °C 3–5 min.

20. Collect using MEF culture medium and pool the eight dishes into a 50 ml conical tube.

21. Centrifuge at $800 \times g$ for 5 min.

22. As cells are spinning, make FM.

23. Aspirate medium off cells and resuspend cells in 10 ml of FM.

24. Add 1 ml of cells to cryogenic tubes, place in Styrofoam container, and freeze at −80 °C.

25. The next day store cryogenic tubes in liquid nitrogen.

3.2 Production of MEF-Conditioned Medium

This protocol should yield approximately 3.36 l of MEF-conditioned medium. Collected medium is stored at −20 °C. When MEF-conditioned medium is thawed for use, add fresh bFGF to 2 ng/ml and pass through a 22 μm filter.

1. Wash two confluent 100 mm dishes containing P3 MEFs with 4 ml PBS each.

2. Add 2 ml 0.05 % trypsin to each dish and incubate at 37 °C for 3–5 min.

3. Collect using MEF culture medium and pool the two dishes into a 50 ml conical tube.

4. Centrifuge at $800 \times g$ for 5 min.

5. Aspirate medium and resuspend cells in 12 ml of MEF culture medium.

6. Plate 1 ml of cells in a 100 mm dish × 12 dishes.

7. Add 9 ml MEF culture medium and gently rock dish to disperse cells evenly.

8. Change medium on all dishes after 2 days

9. When cells are confluent (usually 3 or 4 days), wash each dish with 4 ml PBS.

10. Add 0.05 % trypsin and incubate at 37 °C for 3–5 min.

11. Collect all dishes with 12 ml MEF culture medium and place in 50 ml conical tube.

12. Add an additional 24 ml MEF culture medium to the 50 ml conical tube and centrifuge at $800 \times g$ for 5 min.

13. Aspirate medium and resuspend in 24 ml MEF culture medium.

14. Irradiate cells with 40 Gy (*see* **Note 7**).

15. Count cells with hemocytometer and trypan blue.

16. Plate $4.0–4.5 \times 10^6$ cells per 100 mm dish (typically 12 dishes).

17. Add MEF culture medium to final volume of 10 ml.

18. The next day cells should be confluent, and rinse each dish with 4 ml PBS.

19. Add 40 ml of HESCM to each dish.

20. Next day harvest medium from all dishes into 2×250 ml bottles.

21. Add fresh 40 ml HESCM to each dish.

22. Repeat **steps 20** and **21** for total of 7 days.

3.3 Preparation of Irradiated MEF Stocks in Cryovials

1. Thaw vial of P2 DR4 MEFs by placing vial of cells in 37 °C water bath without submersing the cap. Swirl gently.

2. When no crystals remain, wipe vial with 70 % ethanol and place in cell culture hood.

3. Use a sterile pipette to transfer cells to 50 ml conical tube containing 5 ml MEF culture medium.

4. Centrifuge at $800 \times g$ for 5 min.

5. Aspirate medium and resuspend cells in 10 ml of MEF culture medium.

6. Add 1 ml of cell suspension to 100 mm dish for a total of ten dishes.

7. Add 9 ml of MEF culture medium and gently rock dish to disperse cells evenly.

8. Place cells in 37 °C incubator.

9. Aspirate medium and add 10 ml new MEF culture medium every 3 days.

10. When cells are confluent, aspirate medium and wash eight dishes with 4 ml PBS each.

11. Add 2 ml 0.05 % trypsin to each washed dish and incubate at 37 °C for 3–5 min.

12. Collect using MEF culture medium and pool into a 50 ml conical tube.

13. Centrifuge at $800 \times g$ for 5 min.

14. Resuspend cells in 42 ml MEF culture medium.

15. Plate 1 ml of cells into 100 mm dish×42 dishes.

16. Add 9 ml MEF culture medium to each dish and gently rock dish to disperse cells evenly.

17. For the remaining 2×100 mm dishes, aspirate medium and wash cells with 4 ml PBS.

18. Add 2 ml 0.05 % trypsin to each dish and incubate at 37 °C for 3–5 min.

19. Collect using MEF culture medium and pool into a 50 ml conical tube.

20. Centrifuge at $800 \times g$ for 5 min.

21. As cells are spinning, make fresh FM.

22. Aspirate medium off cells and resuspend cells in 10 ml of FM.

23. Place 1 ml of cell suspension in cryovial, put in room-temperature isopropanol freezing containers, and place containers in –80 °C overnight.

24. The next day store cryogenic tubes in liquid nitrogen.

25. Aspirate medium on cultured dishes and add 10 ml new MEF culture medium every 3 days.

26. When cells are confluent, aspirate medium and wash cells with 4 ml PBS (collect six dishes at a time).

27. Add 2 ml 0.05 % trypsin to each dish and incubate at 37 °C for 3–5 min.

28. Use 8 ml of MEF culture medium to collect each dish and pool three dishes into a 50 ml conical tube.

29. Use 10 ml MEF culture medium to rinse 3×100 mm dishes and add to 50 ml conical tube.

30. Centrifuge both tubes at $800 \times g$ for 5 min.

31. Aspirate medium off 50 ml conical tubes and collect next six dishes.

32. Repeat **steps 19** and **24** until all dishes have been harvested.

33. Resuspend both cell pellets in 10 ml MEF culture medium and combine into one tube.

34. Count cells with hemocytometer and trypan blue.

35. Irradiate cells with 40 Gy (*see* **Note 7**).

36. Centrifuge at $800 \times g$ for 5 min and aspirate medium.

37. Prepare fresh FM.

38. Resuspend cells in freezing medium at 4×10^6 cells per ml (*see* **Notes 8** and **9**).

39. Place 1 ml of cell suspension in cryovial, put in room-temperature isopropanol freezing containers, and place containers in –80 °C overnight.

40. The next day store cryogenic tubes in liquid nitrogen.

3.4 Preparing Irradiated-MEF Plates for iPSCs

1. In sterile hood add autoclaved 0.1 % gelatin to tissue culture dishes as indicated in Table 1.

2. Place dishes containing gelatin in incubator at 37 °C for a minimum of 5 min or maximum of several hours.

3. Thaw MEFs (*see* **Note 10**).

4. Transfer cells from cryovial to 15 ml conical tube with 5 ml pipette.

5. Add 4 ml MEF culture medium.

6. Centrifuge at $800 \times g$ for 5 min and aspirate medium.

7. Cells are resuspended as desired and plated (*see* **Note 11**).

Table 1
Gelatin coating dishes

Culture dish/plate size	0.1 % gelatin added
100 mm	7 ml
60 mm	3.5 ml
35 mm	2 ml
6 Well	1 ml per well
12 Well	0.5 ml per well
24 Well	0.5 ml per well

Table 2
Relative amounts of LV reprogramming vectors

Reprogramming vector	MOI
LV-OCT4	1
LV-SOX2	0.015
LV-LIN28	0.5
LV-NANOG	1

8. Allow MEFs to attach for minimum 8 h; it is best to allow MEFs to attach overnight.

9. Plated MEFs can be used for up to 7 days.

3.5 Generating iPSCs from Fibroblasts/ Mesenchymal Stem Cells Using Lenti and Foamy Viral Reprogramming Vectors

This protocol is based on two previously published papers for lentiviral and foamy viral vector-mediated reprogramming [3, 7].

1. Seed human fibroblasts/MSCs at 2×10^5 cells per well in 6-well plate in MEF culture medium/MSCM.

2. Incubate at 37 °C overnight.

3. Aspirate off medium and add 2 ml fresh medium to each well.

4. For lentiviral infections, add 4 μg/ml polybrene to each well and infect each well with LV vectors at corresponding multiplicity of infection (MOI) (Table 2) (*see* **Note 12**).

   For excisable FV reprogramming vector transductions, infect each well with foamy viral reprogramming vector (ΔΦ53MOSKMETNW) at MOI 1.

5. Prepare two MEF-coated dishes (*see* Subheading 3.4) for each infected well.

6. The next day, wash transduced wells with 2 ml PBS.

7. Add 0.5 ml 0.05 % trypsin to each well and incubate at 37 °C for 3–5 min.

8. Collect each with 4.5 ml MEF culture medium/MSCM and place in 50 ml conical tube.

9. Centrifuge at $800 \times g$ for 5 min.

10. Aspirate medium off conical tubes and MEF dishes.

11. Resuspend transduced cells in 20 ml of the appropriate growth medium.

12. Plate 10 ml of viral transduced cells onto MEFs, two dishes of transduced cells per each well containing MEFs.

13. The next day wash each dish with 4 ml PBS twice.

14. Change medium on all dishes to HESCM.

15. Change medium daily with HESCM for the next 8 days.

16. After 8 days, change medium to MEF-conditioned medium and replace daily until clones have been picked.

17. From days 14 to 20, scan dishes and monitor changing cell morphology using inverted microscope.

18. Between 21 and 30 days after transduction, colonies should be ready to be isolated.

19. One day prior to picking colonies, plate MEFs into 24-well plates. Prepare one well of MEFs for each iPS colony to be picked.

20. Prepare sterile Pasteur pipette hooked cutting tool using Bunsen burner by the following:

    (a) Heat pipette 1/3 distance from end of tip and make a 90° bend in pipette (Fig. 1).

    (b) Allow it to cool and apply more heat near bend. Then pull glass apart to form pointed pipette end (*see* **Note 13**).

    (c) Remove excess glass by tapping with another pipette to generate cutting tool.

21. Wipe dissecting microscope with 70 % ethanol and place into tissue culture hood (*see* **Note 14**).

22. While visualizing colony under dissecting microscope, use pipette to gently cut around colony to mechanically dissociate it from MEFs. It is best to cut colony into pieces (*see* **Note 15**).

23. Once colony has been freed, use P1000 pipettor to collect colony pieces and transfer to a well of a 24-well plate.

24. Repeat **steps 22** and **23** until all desired colonies have been picked (*see* **Note 16**).

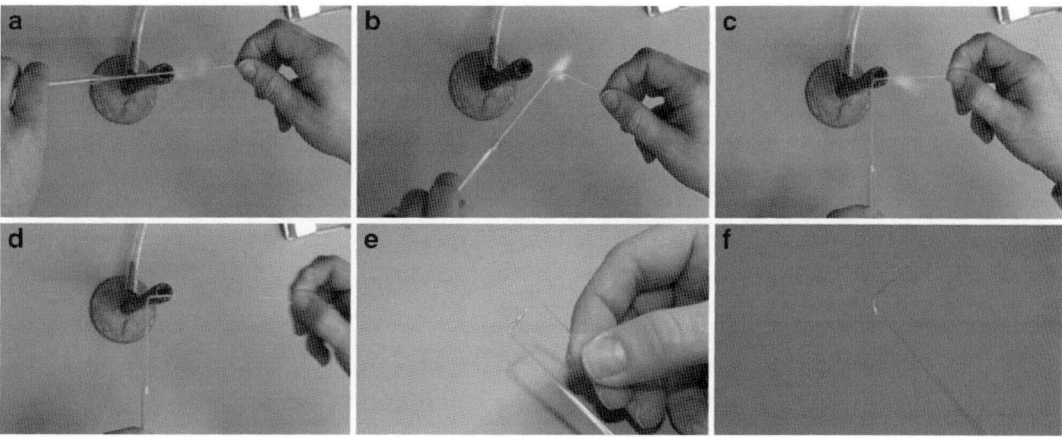

Fig. 1 Creating the cutting tool from a Pasteur pipette. To create the cutting tool to pick iPSC colonies, heat Pasteur pipette over Bunsen burner and make a 90° bend approximately 1/3 distance from the tip (**a**, **b**) and allow to cool. Carefully holding the end, place pipette into flame again distal to the 90° bend, and as the glass softens, quickly pull bend and end away from each other (**c**, **d**). Remove excess glass by tapping with another pipette to generate cutting tool (**e**, **f**)

25. Allow outgrowth of the picked colony (usually 3–5 days) and passage colony into new well of a 24-well plate using dispase (*see* Subheading 3.6).

26. Expand clones by serial passage cells into larger culture dishes to meet laboratory needs.

3.6 Passaging iPSCs with Dispase

1. Aspirate medium off iPSCs.

2. Add dispase (0.5 ml for wells in 24- and 12-well plates, 1 ml for wells in a 6-well plate, 2 ml for a 6 cm dish, 4 ml for a 10 cm dish).

3. Incubate at 37 °C until colony edges start to curl (2–5 min).

4. Aspirate dispase and gently add appropriate amount of wash medium to rinse cells (*see* **Note 17**). Be careful not to dislodge colonies (*see* **Note 18**).

5. Aspirate wash and add 1–4 ml of wash medium.

6. Detach colonies from dish using Pasteur pipette or P1000 for small wells (12- and 24-well plates) and a 5 ml pipette can be used for larger wells and dishes. Try to keep the colonies as large as possible.

7. Spin $200 \times g$ for 5 min at room temperature.

8. Aspirate gently (pellets can be loose, so you can use a 5 ml pipette here).

9. Resuspend in desired volume of HESM. Aliquot cells to MEF dishes containing the rest of the necessary HESM medium volume. Place in incubator.

**3.7 Freezing iPSCs
in Straws**

This protocol is based on the published report by Ware et al. [8].

1. Prepare Bio-Cool III controlled-rate freezer by filling tank with methanol, turning it on, setting the start temperature to –10 °C, setting the speed to 1°/min, setting the end temperature to –33 °C, setting the hold minutes to 600 or greater, and setting the alarm to 0 °C. Press RUN to start cooling to –10 °C (see green light under "start").

2. Put canes with buckets in freezer to cool.

3. Prepare fresh FMs (5 ml).

4. Collect 100 mm dish containing 70–80 % confluent, healthy-appearing iPSCs (1×100 mm dish = 5 straws).

5. Aspirate medium off iPSCs.

6. Add 4 ml of dispase to each dish.

7. Incubate at 37 °C until colony edges start to curl (2–5 min).

8. Aspirate dispase and gently add 4 ml of wash medium to rinse cells (*see* **Note 17**). Be careful not to dislodge colonies (*see* **Note 18**).

9. Aspirate wash and add 4 ml of wash medium.

10. Detach colonies from dish using a 5 ml pipette. Try to keep the colonies as large as possible.

11. Spin $200 \times g$ for 5 min at room temperature.

12. Aspirate gently. Pellets may be loose, so you can use a 5 ml pipette here.

13. Resuspend cells in 1.1 ml FMs.

14. Attach straw adaptor to syringe.

15. Attach sterile, plugged straw to the adaptor.

16. Draw up about 1/2 in. FMs, being careful to avoid cells.

17. Draw up about 1/8–1/4 in. of an air bubble.

18. Draw up most of the straw with cells, about 0.2 ml (mix cells first), but leave 1/2 in. to go.

19. Pull straw out of medium, and then draw up last 1/2 in. to plug. Leave 1/2 in. air at bottom.

20. Place back in sterile package.

21. Repeat **steps 17–21** with the other four straws.

22. Briefly flame bottom of straw and use gloved hand to press melted straw together to seal.

23. Repeat **step 23** on top of straw.

24. Return to sterile package and bring to Bio-Cool III freezer.

25. The time between cell resuspension to placing straws containing iPSCs into Bio-Cool III freezer should be at least 15 min.

26. Bring liquid N2 tank near Bio-Cool III controlled-rate freezer. Make sure that canes are ready with buckets.

27. Place straws in buckets at −10 °C for about 1 min.

28. Cool long forceps in N2, then grab straw(s) with forceps above air bubble, and allow ice crystal to form above the bubble. Then place straws back in bucket in Bio-Cool III freezer.

29. Once all straws are set, press RUN again on Bio-Cool III freezer to start controlled-rate freezing.

30. When frozen, load straws into liquid N2 tanks.

3.8 Freezing iPSCs in Cryovials

1. Thaw the required amount of mFreSR, and store on ice.

2. Prepare FMc, and store on ice.

3. Label cryovials.

4. Prechill isopropanol-freezing containers at 4 °C.

5. Collect 100 dishes of iPSCs (1×100 mm dish = 5–6 cryovials).

6. Aspirate medium from iPSCs.

7. Add 4 ml of dispase to each dish.

8. Incubate at 37 °C until colony edges start to curl (2–5 min).

9. Aspirate dispase and gently add 4 ml of wash medium to rinse cells (*see* **Note 17**). Be careful not to dislodge colonies (*see* **Note 18**).

10. Aspirate and add 4 ml of wash medium.

11. Detach colonies from dish using a 5 ml pipette. Try to keep the colonies as large as possible.

12. Spin $200 \times g$ for 5 min at room temperature.

13. Aspirate gently (pellets may be loose, so you can use a 5 ml pipette here).

14. Gently resuspend the cells in 6 ml cold FMc. Take care to leave the cell aggregates larger than would normally be done for passaging.

15. Transfer 1 ml of cells to each labelled cryovial.

16. Place vials into an isopropanol-freezing container and place the container in −80 °C freezer overnight.

17. The next day store cryogenic tubes in liquid nitrogen.

3.9 Thawing iPSCs from Straw

1. Fill 15 ml conical tube with 5 ml HESM or wash solution.

2. Take straw from liquid N2 and place in a beaker of room-temperature water (dH_2O, tap).

3. Wipe straw with 70 % ethanol.

4. Cut bottom of straw with sterile scissors over waste bin.

5. Cut top of straw over 15 ml tube while holding little bit with plug.

6. Let cells drain into tube.

7. Spin at $200 \times g$ for 5 min at room temperature, resuspend as desired, and plate onto MEF-coated dish.

3.10 Thawing iPSCs from Cryovial

1. Rapidly thaw cells in a 37 °C water bath by gently shaking the cryovial continuously until only a small frozen pellet remains.

2. Remove cryovial from the water bath and wipe with 70 % ethanol.

3. Transfer the cells to a 15 ml conical tube.

4. Add 1.5 ml of warm HESCM dropwise to the tube over 5 min, gently mixing as the medium is added.

5. Add an additional 1.5 ml of warm HESCM dropwise to the tube over 1–2 min.

6. Spin at $200 \times g$ for 5 min at room temperature, resuspend as desired, and plate onto MEF-coated dish.

4 Notes

1. ROCK inhibitor has been shown to block apoptosis of dissociated cultured human embryonic stem cells and thereby increasing survival [9].

2. Lentiviral vectors can be purchased from Sigma. The plasmids are also available from Addgene and each lentiviral vector can be produced as described by Yu et al. [3].

3. The reprogramming plasmid pΔΦ53MOSKMETNW is available from Dr. David Russell's laboratory and the foamy viral vector ΔΦ53MOSKMETNW can be produced as described in Gharwan et al. [10].

4. DR4 MEFs can be purchased from ATCC and Capital Biosciences or they can be isolated from E13 DR4 embryos as described in Manipulating the Mouse Embryo [11].

5. bFGF cannot be refrozen. Once thawed it is best to use the entire aliquot and discard the remainder.

6. DR4 MEFs are resistant to neomycin, hygromycin, puromycin, and 6-thioguanine.

7. MEFs can also be mitotically arrested with mitomycin C by aspirating off the medium on a confluent MEF 100 mm dish. Add 6 ml of MEF culture medium with 10 μg/ml mitomycin C and incubate at 37 °C for 3 h. Remove medium and wash three times with 5 ml PBS. MEFs can be harvested with trypsin and cryopreserved as described in Subheading 3.3.

8. MEFs cannot be stored once thawed. To minimize waste, MEFs can be frozen at higher or lower concentrations for different needs; for example, lower concentration vials can be

used when only a small number of plates or wells are needed for experiments.

9. Alternatively, MEFs can also be frozen in straws. Resuspend cells in FM at 2×10^7 cells per ml. Attach straw adaptor to 1 ml syringe and then fix sterile straw into straw adaptor with plug near adaptor. Draw up a small amount of FM into straw with no cells (~1/2 in.) and then draw in 1/8 in. air to make a bubble spacer. Draw up 0.2 ml of the cell suspension into straw by pulling on syringe plunger leaving a small amount of air at the bottom of the straw. Briefly flame bottom of straw, use gloved hand to press melted straw together to seal, and then repeat on top of straw. Place straws in Styrofoam container, place in freezer at –80 °C overnight, and then store in liquid nitrogen using Plastic goblet cylindrical holder and aluminum cryocanes.

10. Thaw cryovial in 37 °C water bath or straw in 15 ml conical tube containing room-temperature water. For straws, add 5 ml MEF culture medium into 15 ml tube, wipe straw with 70 % ethanol, and then cut bottom of straw with sterile scissors. While holding straw in 15 ml tube, use scissors to cut the top of straw to release cells and then flick straw to drain all fluid.

11. One cryovial (4×10^6 cells) seeds 2–3 100 mm dishes, 4–6 60 mm dishes, or 2 plates (6-well, 12-well, etc).

12. For an MOI of 1 add 100,000 viral particles to 100,000 cells. If titer is 1×10^8 particles/ml, add 1 µl of virus to the cells.

13. Each cutting pipette can be flamed and reused for isolating other iPSC clones. However, after 3–4 uses the tip comes dull, so it is best to make multiple cutting pipettes prior to picking colonies.

14. A dedicated hood with microscope inside is best, but a 70 % ethanol clean microscope can be used. Not all laboratories will be equipped with glass that will accommodate the microscope eyepieces. The dissecting microscope can be placed inside a standard tissue culture hood with the front guard open, but be careful not to contaminate cells while picking colonies.

15. Cut a circle around colony and then make an X through the colony. The colony will be further broken to chunks when being picked up with P1000 pipette.

16. Not all clones will be fully reprogrammed, which is necessary for expansion. It is best to pick as many colonies as possible to maximize the number of isolated clones.

17. DMEM/F12 can be used as wash medium, but HESCM is better. HESCM medium that is greater than 14 days old and cannot be used as culture medium can be used as a wash solution.

18. Dispase is not inactivated by medium, so dilution is required. By carefully rinsing dishes, there is one less spin step.

References

1. Takahashi K, Yamanaka S (2006) Induction of pluripotent stem cells from mouse embryonic and adult fibroblast cultures by defined factors. Cell 126:663–676

2. Takahashi K, Tanabe K, Ohnuki M et al (2007) Induction of pluripotent stem cells from adult human fibroblasts by defined factors. Cell 131:861–872

3. Yu J, Vodyanik MA, Smuga-Otto K et al (2007) Induced pluripotent stem cell lines derived from human somatic cells. Science 318:1917–1920

4. Chan EM, Ratanasirintrawoot S, Park IH et al (2009) Live cell imaging distinguishes bona fide human iPS cells from partially reprogrammed cells. Nat Biotechnol 27:1033–1037

5. Robinton DA, Daley GQ (2012) The promise of induced pluripotent stem cells in research and therapy. Nature 481:295–305

6. Xu C, Inokuma MS, Denham J et al (2001) Feeder-free growth of undifferentiated human embryonic stem cells. Nat Biotechnol 19:971–974

7. Deyle DR, Khan IF, Ren G et al (2012) Normal collagen and bone production by gene-targeted human osteogenesis imperfecta iPSCs. Mol Ther 20:204–213

8. Ware CB, Nelson AM, Blau CA (2005) Controlled-rate freezing of human ES cells. Biotechniques 38:879–880, 882–883

9. Watanabe K, Ueno M, Kamiya D et al (2007) A ROCK inhibitor permits survival of dissociated human embryonic stem cells. Nat Biotechnol 25:681–686

10. Gharwan H, Hirata RK, Wang P et al (2007) Transduction of human embryonic stem cells by foamy virus vectors. Mol Ther 15:1827–1833

11. Hogan B (1994) Manipulating the mouse embryo: a laboratory manual. Cold Spring Harbor Laboratory Press, Plainview, NY

Part II

Molecular Biology

Chapter 6

Profiling Histone Modifications by Chromatin Immunoprecipitation Coupled to Deep Sequencing in Skeletal Cells

Mark B. Meyer, Nancy A. Benkusky, and J. Wesley Pike

Abstract

Chromatin, tightly packaged genomic DNA, is reliant on posttranslational modification of histone N-terminal tails for accessibility of DNA by transcription factors to activate transcription. Each histone modification may denote permissible states for gene activation or repression. As cells undergo differentiation, as they do in the skeleton from multipotential precursors through osteoblasts and into osteocytes, their histone code may be altered to help accommodate these transitions. Here we describe the methodology of chromatin immunoprecipitation (ChIP) coupled to deep sequencing (ChIP-seq) on skeletal cells that have differentiated in cell culture.

Key words ChIP, ChIP-seq, Histone, Bone, MC3T3-E1

1 Introduction

Chromatin immunoprecipitation (ChIP) was originally pioneered in 1985 to investigate direct protein binding to DNA in vivo [1, 2]. Over the past several decades, the assay, now coupled to deep sequencing techniques, has become extremely versatile in determining the location and mechanism for transcription factors, positioning of nucleosomes, and modification of histones, as highlighted by the ENCODE project [3]. Chromatin is able to be densely packed around histone proteins, whose N-terminal regions are exposed and often referred to as histone "tails." Chromatin-modifying proteins are able to facilitate posttranslational modifications on histone tails such as acetylation, methylation, phosphorylation, and deimination to alter the structure of chromatin and ultimately regulate transcription [4]. Several histone tail modifications do occur on the same histone at the same time, the combination of which is referred to as the "histone code" [5].

Jennifer J. Westendorf and Andre J. van Wijnen (eds.), *Osteoporosis and Osteoarthritis*, Methods in Molecular Biology, vol. 1226, DOI 10.1007/978-1-4939-1619-1_6, © Springer Science+Business Media New York 2015

The certain pattern of acetylation or methylation on the same histone tail may indicate a propensity for a chromatin environment to be permissible for transcriptional activation or repression. However, this histone code is not a strict code, rather it facilitates an understanding to guiding principles about histone modifications that indicate transcriptional activation or repression, transcriptional enhancers versus gene promoters or transcriptional elongation [3, 6].

Here we apply the ChIP and ChIP-seq methodology to the investigation of histones in skeletal cells. The pre-osteoblast model of MC3T3-E1 cells allows differentiation into mature matrix forming osteoblast cells within 2 weeks of culture in conditions favorable for differentiation [7]. A cell culture system allows for sufficient material to be grown for ChIP-seq assay. After 2 weeks of differentiation, cells are collected for ChIP assay; however the substantial matrix that is formed during the MC3T3-E1 cell differentiation causes complications in the standard ChIP assay. Outlined below is our procedure for growth of MC3T3-E1 cells into mature matrix forming osteoblasts followed by ChIP assay and finally preparation for sequencing. We have analyzed the histone markers H3K4me1 (enhancer/activation), H3K4me3 (promoter), and finally H3K36me3 (transcriptional elongation) around the osteopontin (*Spp1*) gene as displayed in the final figure. Osteopontin is increased during MC3T3-E1 differentiation and the histone marks demonstrate this through increased levels.

2   Materials

1. MC3T3-E1 osteoblasts (ATCC).

2. Growth medium: MEMα supplemented with 10 % heat-inactivated standard fetal bovine serum and 1 % penicillin-streptomycin from Hyclone (Logan, UT).

3. Differentiation medium: MEMα supplemented with 10 % heat-inactivated standard fetal bovine serum from Hyclone (Logan, UT), 1 % penicillin-streptomycin, 10 mM β-glycerophosphate, and 50 μg/mL ascorbic acid.

4. 2 % Alizarin Red solution: Make with ddH$_2$O. Adjust pH to 4.1–4.3. Check pH if solution is more than 1 month old.

5. Von Kossa silver nitrate solution: Mix 5 g silver nitrate with 100 mL ddH$_2$O.

6. Von Kossa sodium carbonate-formaldehyde solution: Mix 5 g sodium carbonate with 25 mL formaldehyde (37 %), and 75 mL ddH$_2$O.

7. 1.5 % Formaldehyde in 1× PBS.

8. Glycine.

9. PBS.

10. Sucrose cushion buffer: Sucrose 10 %, 10 mM Tris–HCl, pH 7.4, 60 mM KCl, 1 mM EDTA.

11. NCP #1: 10 mM EDTA, 0.5 mM EGTA, 10 mM Hepes, pH 6.5, 0.25 % Triton X-100.

12. NCP #2: 1 mM EDTA, 0.5 mM EGTA, 10 mM Hepes, pH 6.5, 200 mM NaCl.

13. Lysis buffer: 10 mM EDTA, 50 mM Tris–HCl, pH 8.1, 0.5 % Empigen BB, 1 % SDS.

14. IP buffer: 2 mM EDTA, 150 mM NaCl, 20 mM Tris–HCl, pH 8.1, 1 % Triton X-100.

15. ChIP wash #1: 2 mM EDTA, 20 mM Tris–HCl, pH 8.1, 0.1 SDS %, 1 % Triton X-100, 150 mM NaCl.

16. ChIP wash #2: 2 mM EDTA, 20 mM Tris–HCl, pH 8.1, 0.1 % SDS, 1 % Triton X-100, 500 mM NaCl.

17. ChIP wash #3: 10 mM Tris–HCl, pH 8.1, 1 mM EDTA, 250 mM LiCl, 1 % sodium deoxycholate, 1 % NP-40.

18. ChIP wash #4: 10 mM Tris–HCl, pH 8.1, 1 mM EDTA.

19. Elution buffer: 1 % SDS, 0.1 M NaHCO$_3$.

20. Dynabeads (Life Technologies, Carlsbad, CA): Either protein A (Cat #10002D) or protein G (Cat # 10003D).

21. Antibodies—H3K4me1, H3K4me3, and H3K36me3 antibodies were purchased from Millipore at 1 mg/mL concentration (Billerica, MA).

22. QIAgen PCR cleanup kit.

3 Methods

3.1 Skeletal Cell Differentiation

1. Culture MC3T3-E1 cells in growth medium in 10 cm tissue culture-treated dishes (confluent density ~5×10^6 cells) for ChIP assay. For Alizarin Red or Von Kossa staining, cells were cultured in six-well dishes (confluent density ~5×10^5 cells) (*see* **Note 1**).

2. At confluency, switch to differentiation medium for 15 days, replenishing the media every 2–3 days.

3. After 15 days of differentiation, stain a plate of cells with Alizarin Red and Von Kossa as described in **steps 4** and **5** (*see* **Note 2**).

4. Alizarin Red staining (in six-well plate): Aspirate media, and wash cells twice with 1× PBS (2 mL/well). Fix cells with 10 % formaldehyde for 20 min at room temp (2 mL/well). Wash cells twice with ddH$_2$O (2 mL/well), and add 2 mL/well 2 %

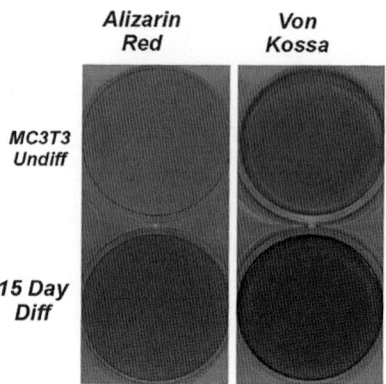

Fig. 1 Alizarin Red and Von Kossa staining for MC3T3-E1 cells undifferentiated (MC3T3 Undiff) and for 15-day differentiated MC3T3-E1 cells (15-day Diff)

Alizarin Red solution for 20 min. Rinse cells 5–6 times with tap water (not distilled water) and air-dry plates, Fig. 1 (*see* **Note 3**).

5. Von Kossa staining (in six-well plate): Aspirate media, and wash cells three times with 1 mL 1× PBS. Add 2 mL of freshly prepared 5 % silver nitrate solution to each well, immediately cover plate with foil, and set aside for 30 min at room temp. Pour out silver nitrate solution, and dab off excess by tapping the plate on a paper towel. Rinse three times with ddH$_2$O (2 mL/well). Add sodium carbonate-formaldehyde solution (2 mL/well) and incubate for 5 min. Rinse plates 4–5 times with tap water (not distilled water). Place 1 mL of ddH$_2$O on each well for storage, Fig. 1 (*see* **Note 4**).

3.2 Chromatin Immunoprecipitation Assay

This assay takes 3 days. **Steps 1–19** are performed on day 1. **Steps 20–30** are performed on day 2. **Steps 31–34** are performed on day 3.

1. Aspirate media from cells. Add 4 mL of 1.5 % formaldehyde in 1× PBS to each plate and shake plates for 15 min at 80 rpm on an orbital style shaker.

2. Add 400 μL of 1.25 M glycine to quench reaction. Continue shaking for 5 min.

3. Aspirate formaldehyde/glycine and wash plates once with 5 mL 1× PBS (4 °C). Swirl and aspirate off the remaining 1× PBS. Add 1 mL 1× PBS (4 °C) back to each plate.

4. Scrape cells from plates and place into a 50 mL conical tube on ice—use cut 1,000 mL tip to move sample. Spin at 1,500 ×g for 5 min in a refrigerated centrifuge (4 °C). Discard supernatant.

5. Resuspend cell/matrix pellet in 10 mL of NCP buffer #1, and swirl to mix. Use a polytron to disaggregate the sample for

30 s. Repeat three times, and place sample on ice for 2 min between repetitions (*see* **Note 5**).

6. Apply sample to top of 13 mL of sucrose cushion buffer.

7. Spin at $300 \times g$ for 20 min in a refrigerated swinging bucket centrifuge (4 °C), aspirate matrix debris off top, retain pellet in about 1 mL buffer, move to 1.7 mL microfuge tube, and spin at $1,500 \times g$ (4 °C) for 4 min.

8. Remove the remainder of buffer, add 1 mL NCP2, resuspend, spin $1,500 \times g$ (4 °C) for 4 min, and discard supernatant. Repeat with 1 mL of NCP2 again (*see* **Note 6**).

9. Remove all residual NCP2 buffer and add 400 µL of ChIP lysis buffer.

10. Sonicate each sample three times for 25 s (until sample clears) with a microtip-style sonic dismembrator. For sonications, keep tip immersed approximately midway in the sample to avoid bubbles. Place sample on ice between sonications to prevent overheating of the sample (*see* **Note 7**).

11. Spin samples for 10 min at $16,100 \times g$ in room-temperature centrifuge to clear cellular debris (due to the SDS concentration, spinning at 4 °C would precipitate the sample).

12. Prepare Dynabeads (A or G) for preclearing. Resuspend slurry well by swirling (Do not vortex beads and never let them dry out). Remove 40 µL of bead slurry per sample and move to new 1.7 mL microfuge tube. Place tube on Dynabead magnet (or similar tube magnet), sit for 30 s to collect, remove storage buffer, and discard. Add 40 µL of ChIP lysis buffer per sample to the beads, take off magnet, resuspend by pipetting, place back on magnet, and let it sit for 30 s. Remove buffer, add 40 µL of ChIP lysis buffer per sample to the beads, take off magnet, and resuspend again. Sample is now ready to be added for protein A or G preclearing.

13. Transfer cellular lysate supernatant to a new tube and add 40 µL of prepared Dynabeads (A or G) to each sample to preclear. Let rotate in cold room for 1 h minimum (*see* **Note 8**).

14. Spin sample with beads at $16,100 \times g$ for 1 min, place on magnet, and move supernatant to a new tube.

15. Spin down again for 1 min, place on magnet, and let it sit for 30 s; this time only retain 380 µL of the sample being careful not to move any beads.

16. Split samples up for each antibody: 100 µL lysate per antibody (histone, IgG control), 2 µL for input samples (2 % of sample volume)—add 298 µL of elution buffer and set aside until the end of day 2. Take 10 µL for DNA sizing—add 290 µL of elution buffer, and set aside at room-temperature until the end of day 2.

17. Add 250 µL of ChIP IP buffer to each sample. Do not add to DNA sizing or input samples.

18. Add 2 µL of each antibody (1 mg/mL concentration) to the appropriate sample (*see* **Note 9**).

19. Incubate on rotator in cold room (4 °C) overnight; place your input samples and DNA sizing at room temperature until the end of day 2 (*see* **Note 10**).

20. At the beginning of day 2, repeat Dynabead preparation for IP as described in **step 12**. Sample is now ready to be added.

21. Add 40 µL of Dynabeads (A or G) to each sample tube and allow to rotate for at least 1 h at 4 °C (*see* **Note 11**).

22. Spin samples at $16,100 \times g$ for 1 min at 4 °C, place on magnet, and let them sit for 30 s.

23. Discard supernatant by pipetting. Be careful not to move any beads.

24. Add 1 mL of ChIP wash #1 to each tube. Move bead/supernatant mix into new tubes, and resuspend fully with a pipette. There may be clumps of beads; pipetting up and down is crucial to remove the clumps (do not vortex) (*see* **Note 12**).

25. Place samples on magnet, let them sit for 30 s, and remove all buffer (can aspirate carefully here).

26. Add 1 mL of ChIP wash #2, remove from magnet, resuspend with pipette, place back on magnet, and let it sit for 30 s.

27. Discard, and repeat with ChIP wash #3, and ChIP wash #4 twice for a total of five washes.

28. At the final addition of ChIP wash #4, spin down samples for 30 s at $16,100 \times g$ before placing on magnet (so the pellets will not dry out for the next step). Remove all buffer with pipette, respin for 30 s max speed, now place on magnet, and remove all residual TE buffer.

29. Add 300 µL of elution buffer and resuspend the pellet by pipetting.

30. Add 12 µL of 5 M NaCl to each tube, mix by inversion, and place in hybridization oven at least 6 h to overnight at 65 °C; do the same with input and sizing samples initially set aside on day 1 (*see* **Note 13**). This is the end of day 2.

31. At the beginning of day 3, spin down samples for 5 min at $16,100 \times g$, room-temp centrifuge, and move supernatant to a new tube—leave beads behind. Repeat spin and place tubes on magnet to ensure that all beads are pulled out of solution. Move supernatant to a new tube.

32. Clean up samples using the QIAgen PCR cleanup kit): Add 1.2 mL of Buffer PB (from the QIAgen PCR cleanup kit) to

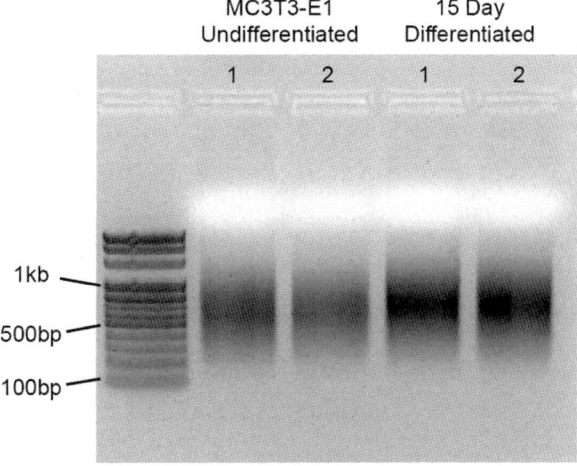

Fig. 2 DNA sizing gel after sonication

each sample, bind the DNA to the columns 750 μL at a time, wash with 750 μL of PE buffer, spin again to dry the column, and elute with 50 μL of TE.

33. Store samples at 4 °C. Use 2 μL of sample for PCR reactions along with appropriate primers to test known regions. Positive control regions are necessary before moving to the next expensive steps. Make a standard curve by diluting the input samples (example: 1:5 serial dilutions).

34. DNA sizing samples: Elute sizing samples in 50 μL water, place at 95–100 °C with lids open for 10 min (boil off residual EtOH), make 0.7 % agarose gel with large width combs, add 15 μL of dye, load as much as possible (45–50 μL) on gel, and take picture after 30–40 min (Fig. 2).

3.3 ChIP-Seq Library Preparation, Sequencing, and Data Analysis

1. ChIP-seq library preparation: We recommend using the NEXTflex ChIP-Seq Kit from Bio Scientific with the ChIP-seq Barcodes following all manufacturers' instructions. Samples may also be processed by a core facility appropriate to the sequencers that will be used for data analysis such as the Illumina HiSeq or GAIIx sequencers.

2. Illumina Hi-Seq or GAIIx sequencing: Samples will need to be processed and sequenced by a core facility. The details of this procedure are beyond the scope of this chapter. Also, these methods may change over time as deep sequencing techniques advance.

3. Data analysis: The most complicated portion of profiling histones is the data analysis. Like the sequencing procedures, data analysis is constantly undergoing revision and optimization as ChIP-seq and high-throughput sequencing evolve. Popular

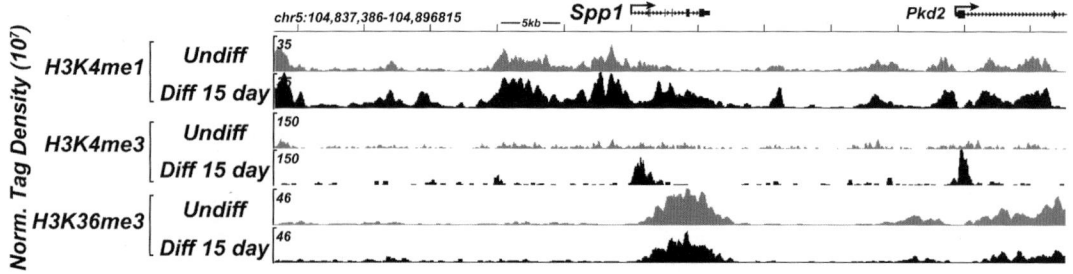

Fig. 3 ChIP-seq tag density profiles for Spp1 (osteopontin) for H3K4me1, H3K4me3, and H3K36me3. Each histone mark is shown in MC3T3-E1 cells undifferentiated (Undiff) and then 15 days after differentiation (15-day Diff). Genomic location (mouse mm9 genome) and scale are indicated in each track, and max height of tag sequence density for the data track is indicated on *Y*-axis. Gene transcriptional direction is indicated by an *arrow* and exons by *boxes*

data analysis techniques include MACS (Model-based Analysis for ChIP-seq) [8], HOMER (Hypergeometric Optimization of Motif EnRichment) [9], and Cistrome Data Analysis [10].

4. Analyzed ChIP-seq data tracks can be visualized using the UCSC Genome Browser in the mouse genome [11] (Fig. 3).

4   Notes

1. We recommend using 5 million cells per histone for ChIP-seq, which equates to 1 or 2 plates of MC3T3-E1 cells per antibody used. If the cells are cultured and available in high quantities, you may consider using 10 million cells per histone ChIP-seq. In general, starting with more material may yield better ChIP-seq results.

2. A 10 cm plate can be used for staining instead of a six-well plate; just scale all the volumes accordingly. This plate will be terminal and should be cultured in parallel with the experimental plates.

3. Alizarin Red plates can be stored dry at room temperature.

4. Von Kossa plates can be stored with a small amount of water in each well, and parafilm wrapped at 4 °C for extended periods of time.

5. After 15 days of culturing, the MC3T3 cells will have a substantial amount of matrix that is very difficult to remove. We utilize a polytron homogenizer to disrupt the cells and matrix. We then collect and buffer exchange with a sucrose gradient buffer. Nuclei can be stained after disruption to ensure that they are still intact. Collagenase digestion has also been tested; however the times needed for complete digestion via collagenase lead to degraded ChIP material.

6. NCP buffer 2 can be repeated several times to remove extracellular debris from the nuclei.

7. Sonication may be completed with a water bath-style sonicator as well. Monitor the sizes of the DNA via the DNA sizing analysis. Ideal DNA sizing would be from 200 to 1,000 bp for the bulk of the DNA. There will be some heterochromatin that will not shear by sonication and may remain at the top of the wells during DNA sizing tests.

8. During the preclearing, if any clumping occurs, which may happen especially with animal tissues, repeat preclear with new Dynabeads until there are no clumps present in the sample.

9. Antibody amount will need to be optimized for each histone marker used. In general, 2 μL of histone marker (at 1 mg/mL concentration) should be enough for most ChIP-seq samples. Note that these volumes are different if one is doing a transcription factor ChIP-seq; in that case, multiply the antibody and cell number by 10. For validated antibodies, please refer to the ENCODE consortium publications [3, 6].

10. Do not place any sample in elution buffer at 4 °C or on ice; the SDS will cause precipitation.

11. Samples can incubate with beads overnight if necessary.

12. Moving samples to a fresh new tube can lower the background.

13. A heat block or water bath can be used for the 65 °C incubation overnight.

Acknowledgements

This research was supported, in part, by grants from NIDDK (DK072281; DK073995; DK074993) and NIAMs (AR045173; AR064424) to JWP.

References

1. Solomon MJ, Varshavsky A (1985) Formaldehyde-mediated DNA-protein crosslinking: a probe for in vivo chromatin structures. Proc Natl Acad Sci U S A 82:6470–6474

2. Solomon C, Sebag M, White JH et al (1998) Disruption of vitamin D receptor-retinoid X receptor heterodimer formation following ras transformation of human keratinocytes. J Biol Chem 273:17573–17578

3. Yavartanoo M, Choi JK (2013) ENCODE: a sourcebook of epigenomes and chromatin language. Genomics Inform 11:2–6

4. Taverna SD, Li H, Ruthenburg AJ et al (2007) How chromatin-binding modules interpret histone modifications: lessons from professional pocket pickers. Nat Struct Mol Biol 14:1025–1040

5. Turner BM (2007) Defining an epigenetic code. Nat Cell Biol 9:2–6

6. Wang Z, Zang C, Rosenfeld JA et al (2008) Combinatorial patterns of histone acetylations and methylations in the human genome. Nat Genet 40:897–903

7. Meyer MB, Benkusky NA, Lee CH et al (2014) Genomic determinants of gene regulation by 1,25-Dihydroxyvitamin D3 during osteoblast-lineage cell differentiation. J Biol Chem 289:19539–19554

8. Zhang Y, Liu T, Meyer CA et al (2008) Model-based analysis of ChIP-seq (MACS). Genome Biol 9:R137

9. Heinz S, Benner C, Spann N et al (2010) Simple combinations of lineage-determining transcription factors prime cis-regulatory elements required for macrophage and B cell identities. Mol Cell 38:576–589

10. Liu T, Ortiz JA, Taing L et al (2011) Cistrome: an integrative platform for transcriptional regulation studies. Genome Biol 12:R83

11. Kent WJ, Sugnet CW, Furey TS et al (2002) The human genome browser at UCSC. Genome Res 12:996–1006

Chapter 7

Identification of microRNAs in Human Plasma

Bram C. van der Eerden, Rodrigo D. Alves, Christel E. Kockx, Zeliha Ozgur, Marijke Schreuders-Koedam, Jeroen van de Peppel, Wilfred F. van Ijcken, and Johannes P. van Leeuwen

Abstract

In recent years, microRNAs (miRNA) have been demonstrated to be present in body fluids and may therefore serve as diagnostic markers for diseases. By characterizing miRNA profiles in plasma, a miRNA signature may potentially be developed as a diagnostic and risk assessment tool for particular (patho)physiological states. This chapter describes the isolation, purification, identification, and sequencing of human plasma miRNAs.

Key words miRNA, Whole-genome sequencing, Plasma, RNA isolation, Human

1 Introduction

There is a great need for improved early diagnosis and risk prediction of osteoporosis, a very common bone-debilitating condition among the elderly, characterized by loss of bone mass and increased bone fragility and fracture risk [1]. A novel group of molecules that may serve this purpose are miRNAs. These are small noncoding RNA molecules that are capable of inhibiting target gene function at the transcriptional or posttranscriptional level. The latter occurs predominantly by binding of the miRNA to the mRNAs of target genes, thereby affecting mRNA stability or inhibiting of translation.

Many studies have shown correlations between the occurrence of tissue miRNAs and cancer incidence and/or severity. For instance, specific miRNA signatures have been described in relation to leukaemia; breast, lung, and hepatocellular carcinomas; and other solid tumors [2, 3]. With the discovery and characterization of miRNAs in different body fluids [4], studies were conducted to determine whether circulating miRNA profiles could be correlated with disease or specific physiological states [5]. Indeed, they turned out to

Jennifer J. Westendorf and Andre J. van Wijnen (eds.), *Osteoporosis and Osteoarthritis*, Methods in Molecular Biology, vol. 1226, DOI 10.1007/978-1-4939-1619-1_7, © Springer Science+Business Media New York 2015

be promising biomarkers for cancer detection and drug-induced liver injury [6, 7]. miRNA profiles in plasma were also correlated to different phases of pregnancy [8]. These studies clearly demonstrate that miRNA expression in body fluids may be related to particular (patho)physiological states and that they may serve as markers or indicators for disease. Our group aims to assess a link between plasma miRNAs and bone metabolism. A previous study suggests that miRNA 133a in circulating monocytes is a potential biomarker for postmenopausal osteoporosis [9]. Given the high metabolic activity within the skeleton, we believe that human plasma is a promising source to screen for miRNA profiles in relation to osteoporotic features, such as low BMD and fractures. In this chapter a detailed description is outlined for the isolation, purification, detection, and high-throughput sequencing of human plasma-derived miRNAs.

2 Materials

2.1 Collection of Human Plasma

1. 6 ml vacutainer plasma collection tubes with spray-coated K_2EDTA.
2. Cryovials, 1 ml.
3. Centrifuge.

2.2 Small RNA Isolation and Purification from Plasma

1. TRIzol LS reagent.
2. Chloroform.
3. Ethanol 100 %.
4. miRvana miRNA isolation kit, without phenol (Ambion).
5. RNase-free water.
6. Centrifuge.

2.3 cDNA Synthesis and PCR

1. Taqman small RNA assays (Applied Biosystems).
2. DEPC water.

2.4 Whole-Genome Small RNA Sequencing

1. Truseq Small RNA Sample prep kit (Illumina).
2. NaOAc, 3 M, pH 5.2.
3. NaOH, 2 N.
4. 5 μm filter tube (IST Engineering Inc).
5. Tris–HCl, 10 mM, pH 8.0.
6. Elution buffer (Qiagen).
7. Novex TBE buffer, 5× (Invitrogen).
8. 6 % Novex TBE PAGE gel, 1.0 mm, 10 well (Invitrogen).
9. Scalpels.
10. DNA 1000 chip (Agilent).

11. Orange G loading dye.

12. Ethanol 100 %, –15 to –25 °C.

13. Ethanol 70 %, room temperature.

14. Gel Breaker tube (IST Engineering).

15. High Sensitivity DNA chip (Agilent).

16. SuperScript II reverse transcriptase with 100 mM DTT and 5× first strand buffer (Invitrogen).

17. T4 RNA Ligase 2, truncated.

18. Human Brain Total RNA (Ambion).

19. Ultrapure ethidium bromide: Dilute to 0.5 µg/ml from a 10 mg/ml stock.

20. XCell Sure Lock Mini-Cell electrophoresis unit (Invitrogen).

21. Decon (cleaning agent; Decon Laboratories Limited).

22. cBot Single Read Cluster Plate (Illumina).

23. Truseq SBS KIT-HS v3 (200 cycles) (Illumina).

24. PhIX adapter-ligated control (Illumina).

25. cBot clustering apparatus (Illumina).

26. HiSeq 2000 Sequencer (Illumina).

3 Methods

3.1 Collection of Human Plasma

1. Obtain informed consent from patients and official approval from local ethics committee for collection of human samples.

2. Collect whole blood in 6 ml vacutainer plasma collection tubes with spray-coated K_2EDTA (*see* **Note 1**).

3. Invert the tube eight times and return it to ice.

4. Within 30 min, centrifuge tubes at $1,750 \times g$ for 10 min at 4 °C to separate out the upper plasma fraction.

5. Distribute the obtained plasma into dry ice-cold cryovials, in aliquots of desired amount, and store at –80 °C.

3.2 Small RNA Isolation and Purification from Plasma

Carry out all procedures at room temperature unless specified otherwise. Wear gloves at all times and perform all steps RNase/DNase free.

1. Thaw 400 µl of previously stored plasma sample and transfer this into a 2 ml Eppendorf tube.

2. Add 3 volumes of TRIzol LS and vortex immediately and again after 5 min. Incubate the mixture for 15 min (*see* **Note 2**).

3. Add 312 µl of chloroform, which corresponds to 26 % of the TRIzol LS volume. Shake vigorously by hand for 15 s and leave it for 3 min.

4. Centrifuge the samples at $12,000 \times g$ for 15 min at 4 °C.

5. Collect the upper, aqueous phase containing the RNA (± 800 μl) into a tube and split this in two new Eppendorf tubes.

6. Repeat **steps 2–5** but by starting with 1.5 volumes of TRIzol LS (600 μl) per tube. Vortex the sample directly and again after 5 min. Incubate the mixture for 15 min.

7. Add 160 μl of chloroform (26 % of 600 μl), shake vigorously by hand for 15 s, and leave for 3 min (*see* **Note 2**).

8. Centrifuge the samples at $12,000 \times g$ for 15 min at 4 °C.

9. Collect the upper aqueous phase of both tubes containing the RNA into one tube (± 800 μl).

10. Add 1.25 volume ($\pm 1,000$ μl) of 100 % ethanol (*see* **Note 3**).

11. Pipet the aqueous phase supplemented with ethanol EtOH in a filter cartridge provided in the mirVana kit. The volume capacity is 700 μl, so the sample has to be loaded in several batches.

12. Centrifuge at $10,000 \times g$ for 30 s or until the solution has passed the filter.

13. Discard the flow-through and wash the column with 700 μl wash solution 1 (provided in the mirVana kit).

14. Centrifuge at $10,000 \times g$ for 30 s. Discard the flow-through and wash the column with 500 μl wash solution 2/3 (provided in the mirVana kit).

15. Centrifuge again at $10,000 \times g$ for 30 s and wash once more with 500 μl wash solution 2/3.

16. Centrifuge at $10,000 \times g$ for 1 min to remove residual fluid. Transfer the filter to new collection tube and add 100 μl of preheated (95 °C) water.

17. Centrifuge at $10,000 \times g$ for 30 s to recover the RNA.

18. Use Nanodrop™ (Thermo Scientific) or a similar approach to obtain an estimate of the total amount of small RNA in your sample (*see* **Notes 4** and **5**). Quantification is required to be able to determine how much volume is required for the cDNA synthesis.

19. Store the isolated and purified RNA at –80 °C until further use.

3.3 cDNA Synthesis and Quantitative PCR

1. Thaw the 5× RT primer from the Taqman small RNA assay kit and template RNA on ice.

2. Prepare the cDNA mixture by adding the following ingredients into a 0.2 ml polypropylene tube or a well from a 96-well plate (total volume is 15 μl):

   (a) 10–100 ng RNA in a maximum volume of 11.1.

   (b) 1.5 μl 10× buffer.

(c) 0.075 µl 100 mM dNTPs (*see* **Notes 6**).

(d) 0.5 µl 50U/µl reverse transcriptase (*see* **Note 6**).

(e) 0.095 µl RNase inhibitor (*see* **Note 6**).

(f) 0.75 µl 5× RT primer (specific for miRNA; can be ordered from Applied Biosystems or other suppliers) (*see* **Notes 6–8**).

(g) 0–11.1 µl DEPC water to adjust to a total of 15 µl.

3. Incubate the mixture in a thermal cycler for 30 min at 16 °C, 30 min at 42 °C, and 5 min at 85 °C and cool it to 4 °C.

4. Dilute the obtained cDNA at least five times by adding 60 µl DEPC water to prepare it for quantitative PCR.

5. Use 1–5 µl of the cDNA for PCR. Initially, use 5 µl of cDNA to determine expression abundance of the specific miRNA. If abundance is high, less cDNA (down to 1 µl) may be used.

6. For quantitative PCRs of miRNAs, prepare the cDNA mixture by adding the following ingredients into a well of a 96-well plate (total volume is 20 µl):

(a) 10 µl of 2× Universal PCR master mix.

(b) 0.5 µl of 20× Small RNA assay (from Taqman small RNA assay kit): It contains a primer for specific miRNA that is delivered together with the RT primer for the cDNA reaction (*see* **Note 9**).

(c) 1–5 µl of cDNA (depending on expression abundance).

(d) 4.5–8.5 µl of DEPC water to adjust to a total of 20 µl.

7. Run the PCR according to standard protocol (1 min at 95 °C and 1 min 1 at 60 °C for 40 cycles) on a thermal cycler.

3.4 High-Throughput Small RNA Sequencing

3.4.1 Ligation of 3′ Adapter

1. Remove the ligation buffer (HML), 10 mM ATP, RNA 3′ Adapter (RA3), and ultrapure water from –15 to –25 °C storage and thaw on ice.

2. Briefly centrifuge the thawed Illumina-supplied consumables at 900 × *g* for 5 s and then place them on ice.

3. Preheat the thermal cycler to 70 °C.

4. Prepare the ligation reaction in a sterile, nuclease-free 200 µl safe-lock PCR tube on ice by adding the following ingredients into the tube (total volume is 6 µl):

(a) 1 µl RNA 3′ Adapter (RA3) (*see* **Note 10**).

(b) 5 µl 1 µg total RNA in nuclease-free water.

5. Gently pipette the entire volume up and down 6–8 times to mix thoroughly, and then centrifuge briefly.

6. Incubate the tube on the preheated thermal cycler at 70 °C for 2 min and then immediately place the tube on ice.

7. Preheat the thermal cycler to 28 °C.

8. Prepare the following mix in a separate, sterile, nuclease-free 500 μl PCR tube on ice by adding the following ingredients into the tube (total volume is 4 μl): Multiply each reagent volume by the number of samples being prepared. Make 10 % extra reagent if you are preparing multiple samples.

   (a) 2 μl 5× HM ligation buffer (HML).

   (b) 1 μl RNase inhibitor.

   (c) 1 μl T4 RNA ligase 2, truncated.

9. Gently pipette the entire volume up and down 6–8 times to mix thoroughly, and then centrifuge briefly.

10. Add 4 μl of the mix to the reaction tube from **step 4** and gently pipette the entire volume up and down 6–8 times to mix thoroughly. The total volume of the reaction should be 10 μl.

11. Incubate the tube on the preheated thermal cycler at 28 °C for 1 h.

12. With the reaction tube remaining on the thermal cycler, add 1 μl stop solution (STP) and gently pipette the entire volume up and down 6–8 times to mix thoroughly. Continue to incubate the reaction tube on the thermal cycler at 28 °C for 15 min, and then place the tube on ice.

3.4.2 Ligation of 5′ Adapter

1. Remove RNA 5′ adapter (RA5) and stop solution (STP) from −15 to −25 °C storage and thaw on ice.

2. Briefly centrifuge the thawed Illumina-supplied consumables at $900 \times g$ for 5 s and then place them on ice.

3. Preheat the thermal cycler to 70 °C.

4. Aliquot $1.1 \times N$ μl of the RNA 5′ adapter (RA5) into a separate, nuclease-free 500 μl PCR tube, with N being equal to the number of samples being processed for the current experiment.

5. Incubate the adapter on the preheated thermal cycler at 70 °C for 2 min and then immediately place the tube on ice.

6. Preheat the thermal cycler to 28 °C.

7. Add $1.1 \times N$ μl of 10 mM ATP to the aliquoted RNA 5′ adapter tube, with N equal to the number of samples being processed for the current experiment.

8. Gently pipette the entire volume up and down 6–8 times to mix thoroughly.

9. Add $1.1 \times N$ μl of T4 RNA ligase to the aliquoted RNA 5′ adapter tube, with N equal to the number of samples being processed for the current experiment.

10. Gently pipette the entire volume up and down 6–8 times to mix thoroughly.

11. Add 3 μl of the mix from the aliquoted RNA 5′ adapter tube to the reaction from **step 12** of Subheading 3.4.1.

12. Gently pipette the entire volume up and down 6–8 times to mix thoroughly. The total volume of the reaction should now be 14 µl.

13. Incubate the reaction tube on the preheated thermal cycler at 28 °C for 1 h and then place the tube on ice.

3.4.3 Reverse Transcription

1. Remove the 25 mM dNTP mix, RNA RT primer (RTP), ultra-pure water, 5× first-strand buffer, and 100 mM DTT from –15 to –25 °C storage and thaw on ice.

2. Briefly centrifuge the thawed consumables to 900 × *g* for 5 s and then place them on ice.

3. Preheat the thermal cycler to 70 °C.

4. Prepare the following mix in a separate sterile nuclease-free 500 µl PCR tube by adding the following ingredients into the tube (total volume is 1 µl): Multiply each reagent volume by the number of samples being prepared. Make 10 % extra reagent if you are preparing multiple samples.

   (a) 0.5 µl 25 mM dNTP mix.

   (b) 0.5 µl Ultrapure water.

5. Gently pipette the entire volume up and down 6–8 times to mix thoroughly, and then centrifuge briefly.

6. Label the tube "12.5 mM dNTP Mix" and then place it on ice.

7. Prepare the following mix in a separate, sterile, nuclease-free 200 µl PCR tube by adding the following ingredients into a well of a 96- or 384-well plate (total volume is 13 µl):

   (a) 12 µl 5′ and 3′ Adapter-ligated RNA.

   (b) 1 µl RNA RT primer (RTP).

8. Gently pipette the entire volume up and down 6–8 times to mix thoroughly, and then centrifuge briefly.

9. Incubate the tube on the preheated thermal cycler at 70 °C for 2 min and then immediately place the tube on ice.

10. Preheat the thermal cycler to 50 °C.

11. Prepare the following mix in a separate, sterile, nuclease-free, 500 µl PCR tube by adding the following ingredients on ice into the tube (total volume is 10.21 µl): Multiply each reagent volume by the number of samples being prepared. Make 10 % extra reagent if you are preparing multiple samples (*see* **Note 11**).

   (a) 5.14 µl 5× First-strand buffer.

   (b) 0.5 µl 12.5 mM dNTP mix.

   (c) 2.57 µl 100 mM DTT.

   (d) 1 µl RNase inhibitor.

   (e) 1 µl SuperScript II reverse transcriptase.

12. Gently pipette the entire volume up and down 6–8 times to mix thoroughly, and then centrifuge briefly.

13. Add the entire mix of **step 11** to the reaction tube from **step 9**. Gently pipette the entire volume up and down 6–8 times to mix thoroughly, and then centrifuge briefly.

The total volume should now be approximately 23 μl.

14. Incubate the tube in the preheated thermal cycler at 50 °C for 1 h and then place the tube on ice (*see* **Notes 12** and **13**).

3.4.4 PCR Amplification

1. Remove the PCR mix (PML), RNA PCR primer (RP1), RNA PCR primer index (RPI1–RPI48), and RNA RT primer (RTP) from –15 to –25 °C storage and thaw on ice.

2. Briefly centrifuge the thawed consumables to $900 \times g$ for 5 s and then place them on ice.

3. Prepare the following mix in a separate, sterile, nuclease-free, 500 μl PCR tube by adding the following ingredients on ice into the tube (total volume is 29 μl): Multiply each reagent volume by the number of samples being prepared. Make 10 % extra reagent if you are preparing multiple samples.

   (a) 25 μl PCR mix (PML).

   (b) 2 μl RNA PCR primer (RP1).

   (c) 2 μl RNA PCR primer index (RPIX).

4. Gently pipette the entire volume up and down 6–8 times to mix thoroughly, then centrifuge briefly, and then place the tube on ice.

5. Add 29 μl of PCR master mix to the reaction tube (with 23 μl) from **step 14** of Subheading 3.4.3.

6. Gently pipette the entire volume up and down 6–8 times to mix thoroughly, then centrifuge briefly, and place the tube on ice. The total volume should now be approximately 52 μl.

7. Amplify the tube in the thermal cycler using the following PCR cycling conditions:

   (a) 30 s at 98 °C.

   (b) 11 cycles of:
        10 s at 98 °C.
        30 s at 60 °C.
        15 s at 72 °C.

   (c) 10 min at 72 °C.

   (d) Hold at 4 °C.

8. Run 1 μl of each sample on a high-sensitivity DNA chip according to the manufacturer's instructions. Figure 1a shows typical results from human brain total RNA (*see* **Notes 14** and **15**).

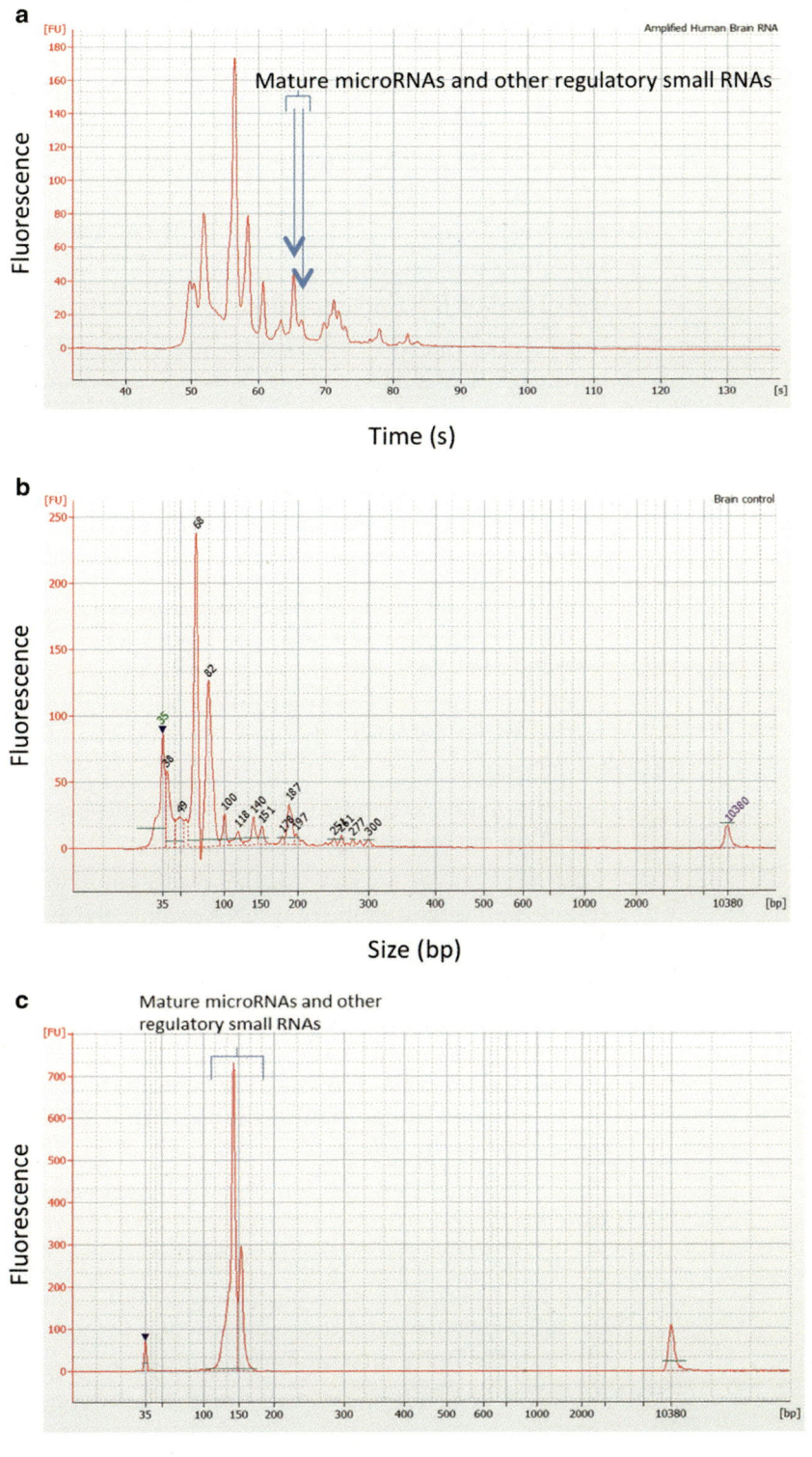

Fig. 1 Sample preparation for next-generation sequencing. (**a**) Bioanalyzer profile of human brain total RNA. (**b**) Human brain total RNA sample trace. The 140 and 151 bp peaks are mature microRNAs with Illumina adaptors. The custom ladder consists of three dsDNA fragments 145, 160, and 500 bp. (**c**) Final sequencing library from a human brain total RNA sample after purification

3.4.5 Gel Electrophoresis

1. Determine the volume of 1× TBE buffer needed. Dilute the 5× TBE buffer to 1× for use in electrophoresis.

2. Assemble the gel electrophoresis apparatus as per the manufacturer's instructions.

3. Mix 2 μl of custom ladder with 2 μl of DNA loading dye.

4. Mix all of the amplified cDNA construct (typically 48–50 μl) with 10 μl of DNA loading dye.

5. Load 2 μl of mixed custom ladder and loading dye in two wells on the 6 % PAGE gel.

6. Load two wells with 25 μl each of mixed amplified cDNA construct and loading dye on the 6 % PAGE gel. A total volume of 50 μl should be loaded onto the gel.

7. Run the gel for 60 min at 145 V or until the blue front dye exits the gel. Proceed immediately to the next step.

8. Remove the gel from the apparatus.

3.4.6 Recover the Purified Construct

1. Pre-chill 100 % ethanol at −15 to −25 °C.

2. Open the cassette according to the manufacturer's instructions and stain the gel with ethidium bromide in a clean container for 15 min.

3. Place the gel breaker tube into a sterile, round-bottom, nuclease-free, 2 ml microcentrifuge tube.

4. View the gel on a Dark Reader transilluminator. Figure 1b shows the human brain total RNA sample trace. The 140 and 151 bp peaks are mature microRNAs with Illumina adaptors. The custom ladder consists of three dsDNA fragments 145, 160, and 500 bp (*see* **Note 16**).

5. Align the razor blade with the top of the 160 bp band of the custom ladder, and then with the bottom of the 145 bp band of the custom ladder. Excise the gel fragment by connecting these cuts on the sides.

6. Place the band of interest into the 0.5 ml gel breaker tube from **step 3**.

7. Centrifuge the stacked tubes at 20,000 × *g* in a microcentrifuge for 2 min at room temperature to move the gel through the holes into the 2 ml tube. Ensure that the gel has all moved through the holes into the bottom tube.

8. Add 300 μl of ultrapure water to the gel debris in the 2 ml tube.

9. Elute the DNA by rotating or shaking the tube at room temperature for at least 2 h. The tube can be rotated overnight, if desired.

10. Transfer the eluate and the gel debris to the top of a 5 μm filter.

11. Centrifuge the filter for 10 s at $600 \times g$ in a benchtop microcentrifuge.

12. Add 2 µl of glycogen, 30 µl of 3 M NaOAc, and 975 µl of pre-chilled –15 to –25 °C 100 % ethanol.

13. Immediately centrifuge at $20{,}000 \times g$ for 20 min in a benchtop microcentrifuge at 4 °C.

14. Remove and discard the supernatant, leaving the pellet intact.

15. Wash the pellet with 500 µl of room-temperature 70 % ethanol.

16. Centrifuge at $20{,}000 \times g$ at room temperature for 2 min.

17. Remove and discard the supernatant, leaving the pellet intact.

18. Dry the pellet by placing the tube, lid open, in a 37 °C heat block for 5–10 min or until dry.

19. Resuspend the pellet in 10 µl 10 mM Tris–HCl, pH 8.5.

3.4.7 Validate the Library

1. Load 1 µl of the resuspended construct on an Agilent Technologies 2100 Bioanalyzer using a high-sensitivity DNA chip.

2. Check the size, purity, and concentration of the sample. Figure 1c shows the final library from a human brain total RNA sample.

3.4.8 Clustering

1. Remove the cBot single read cluster plate and hybridization buffer from –15 to –25 °C storage and thaw in a water bath at room temperature for at least 60 min.

2. Pool six DNA libraries (each library derived from a unique sample with a unique index) to the desired concentration of 2 nM using Tris–HCl 10 mM, pH 8.5.

3. Prepare per sample pool the following mix in a separate, sterile, nuclease-free 1.5 ml nonstick tube by adding the following ingredients (total volume is 10 µl with a final concentration of 1 nM):

    (a) 5 µl 2 nM template DNA.

    (b) 5 µl 0.1 N NaOH.

4. Prepare PhIX library mix in a separate, sterile, nuclease-free 1.5 ml nonstick tube by adding the following ingredients (total volume is 10 µl with a final concentration of 1 nM):

    (a) 1 µl 10 nM PhIX.

    (b) 5 µl 0.1 N NaOH.

    (c) 4 µl elution buffer.

5. Vortex briefly to mix the template solutions and centrifuge for a few seconds at high speed.

6. Incubate the tubes for 5 min at room temperature.

7. Add 490 μl hybridization buffer to the reaction tubes from **step 6**. The final concentration of library stocks and PhIX is 20 pM.

8. Vortex briefly to mix the template solutions and centrifuge for a few seconds at high speed.

9. Add 500 μl hybridization buffer to the reaction tube that contains PhIX.

10. Vortex briefly to mix the PhiX solution and centrifuge for a few seconds at high speed. The final PhIX concentration is 10 pM.

11. Prepare an 11 pM library stock as follows (total volume is 1,000 μl):

    (a) 440 μl hybridization buffer.

    (b) 10 μl 10 pM PhIX stock.

    (c) 550 μl 20 pM library stock.

12. Pipette 120 μl 11 pM library pool into one of the wells of a eight-tube strip. Each well corresponds with one lane of the flow cell.

13. Switch on the cBot apparatus. Wash the cBot one time with 10 ml 5 % Decon and two times with water.

14. Hold the reagent plate by the base, place your other hand on top of the tubes, and then invert the reagent plate ten times to mix the thawed reagents.

15. Centrifuge the plate for 1 min at $250 \times g$.

16. Visually inspect the reagent plate to make sure that no air bubbles exist at the bottom of the tubes.

17. Visually inspect the numbering on the tubes to make sure that they are in the correct order.

18. Remove the non-pierceable red foil of the tube strip in row 10. With one hand, gently hold each end of the tube strip to secure the tubes in the plate. Using your other hand, carefully peel the red foil from the eight-tube strip, taking care not to allow NaOH to spill on your skin or garments, or in your eyes. Discard the foil appropriately.

19. Press down on the tubes to make sure that they are securely seated in the plate and did not become dislodged when you removed the foil.

20. Wash the flow cell with water and dry it with dust-free tissue.

21. Load the reagent plate, the flow cell, the manifold, and the eight-tube strip containing the libraries onto the cBot and start clustering.

22. Remove the flow cell from the cBot when clustering is finished.

23. Wash the cBot with water.

3.4.9 Sequencing

1. Remove the SBS KIT-HS v3 200 cycle kit and the multiplex primer kit from –15 to –25 °C storage and thaw in a water bath at room temperature for at least 90 min.

2. Split the kit in four portions. Place three portions back at –15 to –25 °C storage and use one portion for this sequence run.

3. Remove the flow cell from the flow cell stage on the HiSeq apparatus and replace the gaskets with new gaskets.

4. Place a wash flow cell onto the flow cell stage.

5. Wash the HiSeq with water.

6. Place the sequence reagents into the HiSeq and start to prime the reagents.

7. Remove the wash flow cell and replace it with the clustered flow cell.

8. Start sequencing the flow cell with the following parameters:

   (a) Read 1: 36 cycles.

   (b) Read 2: 7 cycles.

9. Wash the HiSeq with water when the run is finished.

4 Notes

1. It is absolutely essential that the collection tubes for plasma do not contain heparin. It inhibits enzymatic activity, which is required for cDNA synthesis and PCR.

2. TRIzol (in case of cell/tissue samples) or TRIzol LS (developed for liquid samples such as serum/plasma) allows for the extraction of RNA, preserving its integrity during homogenization/lysis steps. Addition of chloroform generates a biphasic aqueous/organic solution allowing the sequential extraction of total RNA, DNA, and protein from the same sample of interest. RNA remains exclusively in the aqueous phase.

3. Ethanol appears to be a more efficient means to recover any-sized RNAs compared to isopropanol (20 nucleotides to several kb) [10]. In addition, isopropanol is less polar than ethanol, which potentially leads to more salt being co-precipitated with the RNA.

4. Quantification of RNA from plasma is not accurate, since small RNAs cannot be accurately measured with the current assays but also because the yields and diversity of miRNAs are low. Be aware that the measured RNA is a reflection of many small RNA moieties in the sample, including miRNAs but also larger RNA molecules, inevitably leading to the question what the precise yield of RNA is from plasma. To circumvent the quantification issue, a good housekeeping miRNA should be taken

along (*see* **Note 8**). This may vary considerably and should be judged with great caution. As a guideline for the quality, the sample can be determined spectrophotometrically by a 260/230 ratio higher than 1.0 and a 260/280 ratio above 1.8.

5. The only accurate means to determine miRNA concentrations is by using the so-called small RNA chips in an Agilent Bioanalyzer (Agilent). This only works well for cell/tissue samples due to abundance and diversity of the miRNAs. Despite many attempts, we and others failed to reliably measure miRNAs in plasma samples.

6. We have optimized the cDNA reaction with 50 % of the recommended volumes of the different ingredients in the reaction mix. The customized RT primer (ordered for each miRNA, separately) was even diluted four times, resulting in a 1:20 dilution versus the 1:5 that is recommended.

7. Up to six RT primers can be added in one RT reaction (0.075 μl/primer) for multiplexing. The advantages of a multiplexed cDNA reaction are that primers for housekeeping miRNAs can be added to the same sample as an internal control (*see* **Note 8**) and costs are reduced.

8. Since quantification of small RNA is problematic, including a good "housekeeping" miRNA in the multiplex cDNA reaction allows for correction of the expression of the miRNA of interest. We routinely use miR-24, miR-93, and U6 snRNA. Another example is miR-16 or different small nuclear/nucleolar RNAs, but other means of normalization have been developed as well [11].

9. We reduced the primer concentration in the PCR reaction by half, without compromising the outcome, thereby reducing costs.

10. The RNA 3′ adapter is specifically modified to target microRNAs and other small RNAs that have a 3′ hydroxyl group resulting from enzymatic cleavage by Dicer or other RNA-processing enzymes. If the amount of miRNAs in your sample is low, like in plasma or other biofluids, the 3′ and 5′ adapters may have to be titrated to prevent interference of non-ligated adapters during the sequencing reaction.

11. RT reaction is used to create single-stranded cDNA.

12. PCR is used to create cDNA constructs based on the small RNA ligated with 3′ and 5′ adapters. This process selectively enriches those fragments that have adapter molecules on both ends.

13. The cDNA is then PCR amplified using a common primer and a primer containing one of 48 index sequences. The introduction of the index sequence at the PCR step separates the indexes from the RNA ligation reaction. This design allows for

the indexes to be read using a second read and significantly reduces bias compared to designs that include the index within the first read. One feature of the TruSeq Small RNA Sample Preparation protocol is to allow use of 48 different index tags to make use of the Illumina multiplexing capability for analysis of directional and small RNA samples.

14. Components of the amplification reaction may interfere with the Bioanalyzer reagents. It may be necessary to dilute the sample before running on the high-sensitivity DNA chip.

15. The bands of the high-sensitivity chip can shift from sample to sample due to an incorrect identification of the marker by the Bioanalyzer software.

16. The 147 nt band primarily contains mature microRNA generated from approximately 22 nt small RNA fragments. A second, 157 nt band containing piwi-interacting RNAs, as well as some microRNAs and other regulatory small RNA molecules, is generated from approximately 30 nt RNA fragments.

Acknowledgment

We thank Tanja Strini for excellent technical assistance. This work was supported by the Netherlands Organization for Scientific Research (NWO; NGI Horizon grant 93511016).

References

1. Das S, Crockett JC (2013) Osteoporosis – a current view of pharmacological prevention and treatment. Drug Des Devel Ther 7: 435–448

2. Calin GA, Croce CM (2006) MicroRNA signatures in human cancers. Nat Rev Cancer 6:857–866

3. Galasso M, Sandhu SK, Volinia S et al (2012) MicroRNA expression signatures in solid malignancies. Cancer J 18:238–243

4. Weber JA, Baxter DH, Zhang S et al (2010) The microRNA spectrum in 12 body fluids. Clin Chem 56:1733–1741

5. Gilad S, Meiri E, Yogev Y et al (2008) Serum microRNAs are promising novel biomarkers. PLoS One 3:e3148

6. Mitchell PS, Parkin RK, Kroh EM et al (2008) Circulating microRNAs as stable blood-based markers for cancer detection. Proc Natl Acad Sci U S A 105:10513–10518

7. Wang K, Zhang S, Marzolf B et al (2009) Circulating microRNAs, potential biomarkers for drug-induced liver injury. Proc Natl Acad Sci U S A 106:4402–4407

8. Chim SS, Shing TK, Hung EC et al (2008) Detection and characterization of placental microRNAs in maternal plasma. Clin Chem 54:482–490

9. Wang Y, Li L, Moore BT et al (2012) MiR-133a in human circulating monocytes: a potential biomarker associated with postmenopausal osteoporosis. PLoS One 7:34641

10. Rio DC, Ares M Jr, Hannon GJ et al (2010) Ethanol precipitation of RNA and the use of carriers. Cold Spring Harb Protoc. doi: 10.1101/pdb.prot5440

11. Kang K, Peng X, Luo J et al (2012) Identification of circulating miRNA biomarkers based on global quantitative real-time PCR profiling. J Anim Sci Biotechnol. doi:10.1186/2049-1891-3-4

Chapter 8

Immunohistochemistry of Skeletal Tissues

Crystal Idleburg, Elizabeth N. DeLassus, and Deborah V. Novack

Abstract

Immunohistochemistry (IHC) is the process of identifying proteins in tissue sections by incubating the sample with antibodies specific to the protein of interest, and then visualizing the bound antibody using a chromogen. Unlike in situ hybridization, which identifies gene transcripts in cells, IHC identifies the products themselves and provides information about their localization within cells (nuclear, cytoplasmic, or membrane) or extracellular matrix. This can be particularly important in the context of bone and cartilage because they contain many cell types as well as matrix components, each with distinct protein expression patterns. As the number of antibodies continues to grow, this technique has become vital for research laboratories studying the skeleton. Here we describe a detailed protocol for IHC analysis of bone and cartilage, addressing specific issues associated with staining of hard and matrix-rich tissues.

Key words Immunohistochemistry, Bone, Cartilage, Decalcification, Fixation, Antibodies, Antigen retrieval

1 Introduction

In both clinical and research studies, histology-based methods are critical for describing phenotypes in patients and in experimental organisms. There are four basic parts to IHC:

(a) Incubation with antigen-specific primary antibody.

(b) Incubation with an enzyme- or a biotin-conjugated secondary antibody.

(c) Detection of secondary antibody via an enzymatic reaction that produces a colored precipitate.

(d) Imaging using standard light microscopy.

However, the tissue collection and processing steps that come prior to IHC are crucial and can greatly affect the quality of IHC. This is particularly true for bone and cartilage where it is necessary to decalcify tissue while maintaining matrix components such as proteoglycans. Therefore careful attention must be paid to

Jennifer J. Westendorf and Andre J. van Wijnen (eds.), *Osteoporosis and Osteoarthritis*, Methods in Molecular Biology, vol. 1226, DOI 10.1007/978-1-4939-1619-1_8, © Springer Science+Business Media New York 2015

each step from tissue harvest and fixation to decalcification and antigen retrieval [1]. Mistakes and overprocessing at any of these steps can damage antigenic epitopes, tissue morphology, or adhesion of tissue to slides, making it difficult to assess morphology and obtain good staining.

1.1 Fixation

Fixation is the process of treating tissue with solutions that preserve gross morphology as well as molecular structures within the tissue and should be started as soon as possible after harvesting the tissue [2, 3]. Penetration of fixative is determined by the size and nature of the tissue of interest. Soft tissues and small pieces of tissue will fix faster than larger or harder tissues. The standard fixative for paraffin embedding is 10 % neutral buffered formalin (NBF). As with most fixatives, this solution preserves tissue by cross-linking the proteins. Therefore, tissues fixed in 10 % NBF usually require antigen retrieval before incubation with primary antibody. Because of the cross-linking action, it is important to avoid over-fixation since this can also quench antigenicity. To ensure proper preservation when working with bone or cartilage, it is necessary to clean away any unwanted soft tissue such as skin and muscle. This allows for fixative penetration in a timely manner and avoids under- or over-fixation. It also makes it easier to orient the bone during embedding.

1.2 Decalcification

To section paraffin-embedded bone, it is essential to soften the tissue before embedding by lowering the calcium content (i.e., decalcification). The duration of decalcification and degree of calcium ion removal are influenced by the solution used. Most commercial solutions are acids, either mineral or organic, and soften bones quickly, but they can easily damage the tissue due to overdecalcification and are generally not compatible with IHC. The most useful decalcifying method for IHC is treatment with 14 % ethylene diamine tetraacetic acid (EDTA) [2–4]. This gentler chelating agent may decalcify hard tissues more slowly but is less likely to damage tissue or affect antigenicity. Even with EDTA, it is important to monitor and optimize the decalcification duration. Failure to do so can lead to overdecalcification, leading to poor morphology and weak IHC staining.

1.3 Antigen Retrieval

Due to the cross-linking action of most fixatives, it is often necessary to unmask antigens before staining [5]. The choice of retrieval method will vary according to the antigens and antibodies used. There are several methods of antigen retrieval but they fall into two main categories, enzyme digestion and heat treatment. Each retrieval method presents its own challenges and optimization for different specimen types is required. Enzyme digestion requires precision in pH and duration of treatment because different tissues will digest at different rates. The challenge in heat retrieval is in treating the tissue long enough to ensure antigen retrieval without causing it to lift off from the slide, which is a common problem when working with cartilage and bone.

1.4 Data Analysis

To accurately interpret staining it is important to know the standard morphology and staining patterns in the tissue of interest. Textbooks on histology, pathology, and developmental biology can be good resources when learning how to interpret IHC data. The first priority is to determine whether the staining is specific or nonspecific ("background"). Having both negative and positive controls is crucial in making this determination. Negative control slides can be generated in two ways: slides are incubated with no primary antibody or slides are incubated with isotype- and species-matched immunoglobulin [5, 6]. Negative controls without primary antibody ("no primary" control) are usually acceptable; the isotype control is the gold standard because it is possible to see interactions between nonimmune immunoglobulins (or serum) from one species and target tissues from another. The "no primary" control does not use any reagents from the primary antibody host and will lack this type of background that could confound your results. Ideally, control slides should have no staining at all. However, some background is often unavoidable, and thus the negative control slides must be directly compared to the test slides in similar areas to demonstrate specificity.

Other important factors to consider are which tissues, cells, or organelles are stained and whether staining patterns make physiological sense based on known molecular pathways. Positive control slides are very useful here, although different tissue types may have quite different staining patterns. Complementary techniques such as in situ RNA hybridization, which identifies gene expression in specific cells, laser capture microdissection with RNA analysis, or tissue fractionation with protein or RNA analysis can also be used to verify and complement IHC findings.

2 Materials

1. Phosphate-buffered saline (PBS).

2. Citrate buffer, pH 6: Make 0.1 M stock solutions of citric acid and trisodium citrate. To 450 mL distilled deionized water (ddH$_2$O) add 9 mL of citric acid stock solution and 41 mL of sodium citrate stock solution. The pH of this final solution should be about 6.0 ± 0.1.

3. 10 % Neutral buffered formalin (NBF).

4. Paraformaldehyde (PFA) can be purchased as a 16 % stock and diluted to a 4 % working solution. Making your own from powder is hazardous, and respiratory precautions must be taken.

5. Peroxidase block (3 % H_2O_2 in methanol): dilute 25 mL 30 % H_2O_2 to a final of 250 mL in 100 % methanol chilled at –20 °C (*see* **Note 8**).

6. Color Frost Plus slides.

7. Vectastain ABC Kit (Vector Labs).

8. DAB Chromogen (Biocare).

9. 14 % Free acid EDTA, pH 7.2 (EDTA decalcification buffer): Mix 140 g EDTA free acid with 700 mL ddH_2O. While stirring, slowly add 30 mL of ammonium hydroxide at 30 min intervals 3 times (for a total of 90 mL ammonium hydroxide). Check the pH. EDTA will not dissolve until pH is close to 7.2. If not up to 7.2, add the remaining 10 mL ammonium hydroxide dropwise to get to pH 7.2 while constantly stirring. Add ddH_2O for a final volume of 1 L. It is critical that this solution is made properly. If the pH goes above 7.4, do not attempt to correct with HCl—just start over.

10. Methanol.

11. Graded ethanols (30 %, 50 %, 70 %): It is least expensive to dilute from a purchased 70 % stock, but 95 % can also be used. These concentrations do not have to be very exact. Adding about 50 or 70 mL of 70 % ethanol and diluting up to 100 mL in ddH_2O are sufficient.

12. Xylene.

13. Coplin jars.

14. Humidity chamber: Any container with a lid can be lined with damp paper towels to make one, and several companies sell them.

15. Mounting medium, xylene compatible such as Richard-Allan Scientific™ Mounting Medium (Thermo).

16. Proteinase K in 10 mM Tris–HCl, pH 7.4–8.0: Make a 10 mg/mL Proteinase K (Roche) stock solution in ddH_2O. 1 M Tris–HCl pH 8.0 is commercially available. Dilute 1 M Tris–HCl stock solution at 1:100 dilution (10 μL/mL) to make a 10 mM Tris–HCl diluent solution. To 1 mL of this diluent solution, add 1 μL of the Proteinase K stock solution to get a final concentration of 10 μg/μL of Proteinase K.

3 Methods

3.1 Tissue Preparation

1. Immediately after dissection, fix bones in 10 % neutral buffered formalin or 4 % paraformaldehyde for 24–72 h at room temperature. Fixative volume should be 15–20 times tissue volume. To ensure complete penetration, tissue should be agitated on a shaker during fixation (*see* **Note 1**).

2. Rinse tissue in PBS or ddH$_2$O six times, 15 min each.

3. Decalcify in 14 % free acid EDTA, pH 7.2, with rocking, changing solution daily (on weekdays only is OK). The number of days required for decalcification of mouse bones is as follows (*see* **Note 2**):

    (a) Embryo > E17.5: 1–2 days.

    (b) Postnatal days (P) 1–4: 3 days.

    (c) P5-P10: 4–5 days.

    (d) P10-P21: 7–10 days.

    (e) Adults: 10–14 days.

4. Rinse tissue in PBS or ddH$_2$O six times, 15 min each, to stop the decalcification process (*see* **Note 3**).

5. Dehydrate the tissue through a series of ethanol solutions, with rocking:

    (a) 30 % ethanol for 15 min.

    (b) 50 % ethanol for 15 min.

    (c) 70 % ethanol for 15 min.

6. Place tissue in the tissue processor for dehydration, clearing, and infiltration before embedding. Typically, a 4-h processing program works well for most machines with mouse long bones (*see* **Note 4**).

7. When processing is complete, the bones are embedded in paraffin. It is important to determine the plane of interest before this point in order to orient the tissue properly.

8. Tissue sections are then cut at 5 μm using a microtome, floated onto a 45 °C with ddH$_2$O bath and placed on color frost slides (*see* **Note 5**).

9. Slides are dried at room temperature overnight. After overnight drying, slides can be stored or processed further (*see* **Note 6**).

3.2 **IHC**

1. Heat slides in a 55 °C oven for 1 h (*see* **Note 7**).

2. Incubate slides in xylene 3 × 5 min.

3. Incubate slides in 100 % ethanol 3 × 3 min.

4. Incubate slides in 95 % ethanol 2 × 3 min.

5. Incubate slides in 70 % ethanol 1 × 3 min.

6. Incubate slides in 50 % ethanol 1 × 3 min.

7. Incubate slides in 30 % ethanol 1 × 3 min.

8. Rinse in ddH$_2$O water (ddH$_2$O) 3 × 5 min.

9. Do not let the slides dry out after this point. Incubate slides in peroxidase block for 10 min (*see* **Note 8**).

10. Rinse slides once in ddH$_2$O (2–3 dips) and then wash in 1X PBS 3 × 5 min. Start the antigen retrieval process by incubating

slides in citrate buffer in a covered Coplin jar at 55 °C overnight (*see* **Note 9**).

11. Rinse slides in PBS 3 × 5 min.

12. Block endogenous biotin with avidin/biotin block according to the manufacturer's instructions. We find that this is important in skeletal tissues.

13. Incubate in 10 % serum diluted in PBS for 60 min at room temperature in humidified chamber (*see* **Note 10**).

14. Drain off serum solution. Do not rinse slides or let the slides dry completely.

15. Incubate in primary antibody diluted with 1.5 % serum overnight at 4 °C or for 1 h at room temperature in humidified chamber. Depending on the size of your tissue, you will need 50–200 μL of antibody solution. Cut a piece of parafilm the same size as the slide and float this on top to retain the antibody over the tissue, taking care not to have any bubbles. Do not use a glass or plastic cover slip (*see* **Note 11**).

16. Rinse slides 3 × 5 min in PBS.

17. Incubate sections in biotinylated secondary antibody for 30 min, following data sheet from the manufacturer for dilutions (*see* **Note 12**). You do not need to use the parafilm for this shorter incubation, but make sure that the tissue is covered with the solution. Do not allow the tissue to dry or you will get very high background.

18. Rinse slides 3 × 5 min in PBS.

19. Prepare ABC solution as per the manufacturer's instructions and incubate with slides for 30 min.

20. Prepare DAB substrate. (*see* **Note 13**).

21. For developing the slides you will need a light microscope. Lay out all your reagents—the substrate solution, several Coplin jars with water to stop the substrate reaction, and slides should all be easy to reach. Some reactions take as little as 30 s before developing background, so there is little margin for error at this point.

22. Place your positive (+ve) and negative (−ve) control slides on the microscope stage and add a drop of substrate solution to each. The ideal time interval will give you the most intense staining in your +ve control without giving any staining in the −ve. The maximum staining time should be 5 min or less. Place the slides in the extra Coplin jars of ddH$_2$O to stop the reaction. Do not return these slides to jars with undeveloped slides because this will start the substrate reaction prematurely.

23. Develop the remainder of the slides one at a time at the optimal time determined in **step 22**. Once a slide has developed put it in the extra Coplin Jar with ddH$_2$O.

24. Rinse slides well in ddH$_2$O.

25. Counterstain the slides in Harris hematoxylin for 30 s to 1 min [7].

26. Wash in running tap distilled water for 10 min.

27. Dehydrate and clear through two changes of 95 % ethanol, and three changes each of 100 % ethanol and xylene.

28. Add cover slip with mounting medium. In a fume hood, place a drop or thin line of mounting medium on the edge of the cover slip on the benchtop and touch it with the edge of an inverted slide at a 45° angle, and gently bring it down onto cover slip. Avoid bubbles under the cover slip (*see* **Note 14**). Wipe the excess xylene and mounting medium from the underside of the slide with gauze or Kimwipe prior to viewing under microscope. Allow slides to dry and xylene to evaporate in a fume hood.

4 Notes

1. For example, 1–2 mouse femurs and/or tibia should be placed in a 15 mL tube with at least 10 mL fixative. Most tissues will be properly fixed in 24 h, but large bones, such as from rabbits, might require longer fixation and larger containers. However, antigenicity can be reduced with longer fixation, so optimization of fix time may be needed.

2. The first time you perform this procedure with new samples, include a test bone of the same type as you will analyze in the decalcification and use this one to bend and compress. A fully decalcified bone should bend easily and not break. Kits to determine complete decalcification can be purchased (eg. Newcomer). Do not bend your actual samples as this will affect morphology, particularly of marrow elements.

3. Total rinse time should be about 2 h.

4. First step in processor should be 70 % ethanol. Whole-bone specimens from larger animals may require 6–8-h processing times.

5. Slides can be checked using light, dark-field, or phase microscopy at this point for proper plane of section.

6. Do not skip this step (i.e., do not go straight to heating slides at 55 °C). The tissue is likely to fall off the slides during staining if the specimens are not dried properly.

7. Alternatively slides may be baked overnight at 55 °C.

8. Start with 10 min, and extend if background is high on negative controls. The 30 % hydrogen peroxide can also be diluted in PBS instead of cold methanol. In addition, there are commercial peroxidase block alternatives such as Biocare 1, which may be preferable because they have shorter incubation times.

9. Slides can also be heated to 95 °C in citrate buffer for 10 min, followed by cooling in hot buffer for 15 min. However, over-night citrate buffer treatment is preferable to high heat because it preserves tissue morphology better. If the high heat method is used, make sure that the buffer does not come to a full boil as this will cause the tissue to fall off the slide. Other alternative retrieval methods include enzymatic digestion at 37 °C with Proteinase K (10 ug/mL in 10 mM Tris–HCl pH 7.4–8.0 for 20 min) or hyaluronidase (1 % in PBS for 30 min). Avoid using reagents generated in donkeys (serum or antibodies) when using hyaluronidase, because it increases background staining. In addition some antigens do not require antigen retrieval. This is a step that must be optimized for each antigen.

10. Blocking and primary antibody incubation serum should be from the same species as the secondary antibody (i.e., if the secondary antibody is goat anti-rabbit then goat serum should be used to block slides).

11. Data from the antibody manufacturer are good sources for determining the primary and secondary antibody concentra-tions to use. However, users may have to run serial dilution experiments to determine the optimal concentration for spe-cific tissue/antibody combinations.

12. Alternatively, incubate in secondary antibody conjugated to horseradish peroxidase, diluted in 1.5 % serum for 30 min at room temperature. If you do this, then skip **step 19** and go straight to **step 20**.

13. We usually use DAB solution from Biocare, although other chromagens are available. DAB generates a brown precipitate, and is very mutagenic. Take care to use gloves and follow the manufacturer's instructions for handling and disposal.

14. You can use gentle pressure to push small bubbles to the edge of the cover slip. If the bubbles are very large, you probably did not use enough mounting medium. Put the whole slide with the cover slip back into xylene to float off the cover slip and start over. If you try to pry off the cover slip, you are likely to damage the tissue.

References

1. Bord S (2003) Protein localization in wax-embedding and frozen sections of bones using immunohistochemistry. Method Mol Med 80: 237–247

2. Carson F, Hladik C (2009) Histotechnology: a self instructional text. American Society for Clinical Pathology Press, Chicago

3. Sheehan DC, Hrapchak BB (1980) Theory and practice in histotechnology, 2nd edn. The C. V. Mosby Company, St. Louis

4. Hao Z, Kalscheur VL, Muir P (2002) Decalcification of bone for histochemistry and immunohistochemistry procedure. J Histotechnol 25: 33–37

5. Battifora H (1999) Quality assurance issues in immunohistochemistry. J Histotechnol 22: 169–175

6. Watkins S (2000) Immunohistochemistry. In: Ausubel FM, Brent R, Kingston RE, Moor DD, Seidman JG, Smith JA, Struhl K (eds) Current protocols in molecular biology, vol 2. Wiley, New York, Supplement 7 Unit 14.6

7. Allen TC, Sobin LH (1992) Harris hematoxylin and eosin procedure. In: Prophet EB, Mills B, Arrington JB (eds) Laboratory methods in histotechnology. Armed Forces Institute of Pathology, Washington, DC, pp 56–57

Part III

Biomechanics and Imaging

Chapter 9

In Vivo Axial Loading of the Mouse Tibia

Katherine M. Melville, Alexander G. Robling, and Marjolein C.H. van der Meulen

Abstract

Noninvasive methods to apply controlled, cyclic loads to the living skeleton are used as anabolic procedures to stimulate new bone formation in adults and enhance bone mass accrual in growing animals. These methods are also invaluable for understanding bone signaling pathways. Our focus here is on a particular loading model: in vivo axial compression of the mouse tibia. An advantage of loading the tibia is that changes are present in both the cancellous envelope of the proximal tibia and the cortical bone of the tibial diaphysis. To load the tibia of the mouse axially in vivo, a cyclic compressive load is applied up to five times a week to a single tibia per mouse for a duration lasting from 1 day to 6 weeks. With the contralateral limb as an internal control, the anabolic response of the skeleton to mechanical stimuli can be studied in a pairwise experimental design. Here, we describe the key parameters that must be considered before beginning an in vivo mouse tibial loading experiment, including methods for in vivo strain gauging of the tibial midshaft, and then we describe general methods for loading the mouse tibia for an experiment lasting multiple days.

Key words Bone, Mechanical loading, Tibia, Mouse, Anabolic bone formation

1 Introduction

In the field of bone metabolism, considerable interest exists in elucidating new anabolic pathways that can be targeted therapeutically to improve bone mass and strength. The dysregulation of certain bone-active signaling pathways, manifest in numerous human diseases of bone metabolism as altered bone mass, size, and strength, has shed light on the mechanisms of normal skeletal homeostasis. More importantly, these observations provide insight into viable molecular targets that can be manipulated in otherwise healthy patients to achieve a therapeutic outcome. Recent efforts in skeletal biology have focused on uncovering new anabolic, rather than anti-catabolic, pathways that can be manipulated to improve bone mass in skeletally fragile individuals. In addition, certain skeletal diseases have yielded targets for anabolic action in bone (e.g., hyperostosis corticalis, sclerosteosis). However, a much

Jennifer J. Westendorf and Andre J. van Wijnen (eds.), *Osteoporosis and Osteoarthritis*, Methods in Molecular Biology, vol. 1226, DOI 10.1007/978-1-4939-1619-1_9, © Springer Science+Business Media New York 2015

more ubiquitous mechanism of bone formation and accrual, that is not based on disease yet is incredibly anabolic, is available for therapeutic discovery. That mechanism is mechanotransduction, the process by which bone responds and adapts to its mechanical environment by adjusting tissue mass, architecture, and material properties.

Repeated increased loading, such as occurs with exercise, has the propensity to induce new bone formation. Conversely, when loads are reduced during conditions such as bed rest, neuromuscular paralysis, or spaceflight, bone mass is lost in the weight-bearing bones. Despite its anabolic potential, our understanding of the cellular and molecular mechanisms that govern this adaptive process is far from complete. To study this process systematically, and eventually identify the anabolic mechanisms involved, reliable, meaningful, well-characterized, and reproducible physiologic models of mechanical loading are crucial, preferably in intact animals. Toward this end, a number of animal-loading models have been developed, including rodent exercise studies, rodent whole-body vibration, and in vivo loading models such as tibial four-point bending, rodent ulnar axial loading, and mouse tibial axial loading [1–6]. An advantage of in vivo mechanical loading models is that controlled, repeated mechanical forces are applied to the skeletal site of interest. In contrast, exercise studies are associated with a mechanical environment that is much more difficult to quantify and is less well controlled.

One in vivo loading model that has been met with broad appeal is the mouse tibial axial loading model. This model applies cyclic, physiologically relevant loads to one tibia while using the contralateral tibia as an internal control [3, 7]. This model has several advantages, including the use of the mouse, and the presence of substantial volumes of cortical and cancellous bone. The mouse is a valuable animal model because of the opportunity to study genetic manipulations, including congenic, transgenic, knockout, and knock-in mice. These genetic models can provide critical insights into the underlying mechanisms involved in mechanotransduction. The mouse tibia can provide information about the skeletal response to applied loads across several bone envelopes: cancellous, periosteal, and endocortical.

This chapter describes general methods for cyclic loading of the mouse tibia. The loading can be performed using a load-controlled mechanical testing system or a custom loading device with Labview software. The basic protocol in our laboratories involves loading groups of mice under isoflurane anesthesia for multiple days, and the procedures described are generally applicable and can be modified to suit an investigator's particular goals. Before beginning a loading experiment, a number of items must be considered. Loading protocols reported in the literature use a variety of different parameters including number of loading sessions per week, number of loading cycles per day, and characteristics of the load waveform including the loading frequency, loading rate, and inclusion of rest periods [8, 9]. Maximum or peak compressive load must also be determined prior to loading by using in vivo strain gauging techniques to measure bone stiffness at the tibial midshaft. Furthermore, before loading experiments are under way, a sham loading experiment must be performed to confirm the lack of systemic effects in any particular laboratory setup. These considerations are first described, followed by a general outline of the strain gauging procedures and in vivo axial tibial loading methods.

Although not the focus of this chapter, before beginning an experiment, relevant outcome measures must be chosen. This choice will affect experimental design, number of animals, and experiment duration. Common outcome measures include gene expression via qPCR, bone geometry and morphology via micro-computed tomography, dynamic histomorphometry via injection of bone-seeking fluorescent labels prior to sacrifice, protein and/or RNA localization via immunohistochemistry or in situ hybridization, mechanical testing, serum measurements via ELISA or RIA, body and organ masses, and many others.

2   Materials

2.1   Animal Model Selection

1. Select mouse strain. The choice of background strain for mouse axial tibial loading will depend on a number of factors. The amount of cancellous bone in the tibial metaphysis varies with mouse strain, as do cortical bone mass, bone mineral density, bone shape, and bone strength [10–14]. Tibia length and mouse size are also items to consider. Furthermore, some mouse strains are more mechanoresponsive than others [15, 16].

2. Select wild-type or genetically modified mice. Depending on the research question, genetically modified mice may help identify whether the response to loading depends on the absence, presence, overexpression, or modification of a particular gene or set of genes.

3. Select appropriate sex. The research question being asked will guide the decision regarding the use of male or female mice (or both). For example, models of postmenopausal osteoporosis are usually performed in female mice, particularly if ovariectomy will be used. Models of osteoarthritis usually use male mice because of the chondroprotective effect of estrogen [17]. Many individual genes or larger quantitative trait loci (QTL) are associated with sex-specific effects, so when dealing with a novel gene or pathway with no a priori knowledge of sex interaction, males and females should both be studied.

4. Select mouse age. Again, this choice depends on the research question. Growing animals are still accruing bone mass, until around 16–24 weeks of age, when peak bone mass is reached, although the specific age varies with bone site and mouse strain [11, 14]. Aged mice are usually in a state of bone loss [18]. Mice that have just reached skeletal maturity (e.g., 16 weeks of age) are often used for tibia loading because the skeleton is still young enough to elicit a robust anabolic response to mechanical stimulation. At the same time, the appositional growth on the periosteal surfaces has been reduced to very low levels. This latter attribute allows for a less complicated interpretation of the load-induced bone formation effects observed in the loaded limb. At this age, the anabolic response is almost exclusively a result of loading, rather than a combined function of growth and enhanced mechanical input (as occurs in loaded growing bone).

2.2 Select Appropriate Controls

1. Sham controls. A separate experiment must be performed to ensure that tibial loading does not cause systemic effects, which have been both confirmed and refuted in the literature [19, 20]. Confirm that paired contralateral control limbs from loaded mice are not different from control limbs obtained from separate non-loaded animals. This experiment should contain two groups of mice for an experimental duration corresponding to that of the planned in vivo tibial loading experiments. The first group of mice should have one tibia loaded while the contralateral limb is used as an internal control. The second group should be put under anesthesia and have one tibia placed in the loading device for the duration of loading just as the first group, but the tibia should not actually be loaded during the experiment (sham loading). If the results from the two sets of control limbs are similar, then paired contralateral limbs are appropriate controls.

2. Paired controls. If no systemic effects are present, the contralateral, unloaded limb is often used as the control tibia, to which all measurable outcomes will be compared in determining bone's anabolic response to mechanical loading.

2.3 Strain Gauging Materials (When Not Specified, Materials Can Be Ordered from Fisher Scientific or Similar Supplier)

1. 60/40 tin/lead solder, 0.022 in. diameter (Multicore Solders, Westbury, NY).

2. Three-conductor cable (Vishay Micro-Measurements, Wendell, NC, Cat# 336-FTE).

3. Soldering iron (GC Electronics, Rockford, IL, Model# 12-070).

4. Dissecting microscope with light source.

5. Dissecting curved jeweler's microforceps (Fisher Scientific, Cat# 08-953F).

6. Standard capacity wire stripping system (American Beauty, Clawson, MI, Model# 10503).

7. Tip tinner (MG Chemicals, Burlington, Ontario, Cat# 4910-28G).

8. Rosin Soldering Flux (Radio Shack).

9. Single element strain gauges (Vishay Micro-Measurements, Cat# EA-06-015LA-120).

10. Scalpel holder and #15 scalpel blades.

11. Isopropyl alcohol.

12. Clear tape.

13. Index cards for gauge preparation.

14. First coat: M Bond Adhesive Resin Type AE (Vishay Micro-Measurements).

15. Catalyst for first coat: M Bond Type 10 Curing Agent (Vishay Micro-Measurements).

16. Second coat: M Coat D (Vishay Micro-Measurements) (store in refrigerator).

17. Third coat: M Coat A (Vishay Micro-Measurements) (store in refrigerator).

18. Weigh boats in which to mix the first coat with the catalyst.

19. Cotton swabs to apply isopropyl alcohol.

20. Wooden applicator sticks to apply coat coverings.

21. Eye dropper or transfer pipettes.

22. Xylene, to thin third coat if needed.

23. Toluene, to thin second coat if needed.

24. Plugs for wires to connect gauge to computer or data acquisition device (Digi-Key, Thief River Falls, MN, Part# A26528-40-ND).

25. 1-, 3-, or 5-min curing epoxy.

26. Digital multimeter.

27. Strain conditioning hardware including bridge excitation, Wheatstone bridge circuit, and signal amplification and filtering. Integrated systems are produced by Vishay Micro-Measurements and National Instruments LabView board (Part #'s 781156-01, 779521-01, 194738-01, 779012-01).

2.4 Surgical Supplies

1. Surgical tools including scissors, small scalpels and blades, jeweler's forceps, periosteal elevator, and small-tooth forceps.

2. Small gauze.

3. Small animal razor.

4. Calipers.

5. Cotton swabs.

6. Methyl ethyl ketone.

7. Cyanoacrylate tissue adhesive.

2.5 Loading Materials

1. Loading device with actuator, calibrated load cell (or similar).

2. Computer with connections for loading hardware and electronics.

3. If using custom loading device, signal conditioning hardware for data acquisition from load cell with Labview software for tibial loading (or similar) (*see* **Note 1**).

4. Loading configuration files to input loading parameters.

5. Wooden cylindrical rod (~17 mm length) from long cotton swab handle (Fisher Scientific, #23-400-118) for loading program test (*see* **Note 2**).

2.6 Mouse Care Materials

1. Rodent cages with food, enrichment (such as a shelter, PVC pipe, running wheel, or hardwood block), nesting material, and water.

2. Rodent anesthesia induction chamber.

3. Mouse anesthesia nose cone.

4. Isoflurane anesthesia machine with tubing attached to anesthesia chamber and mouse nose cone simultaneously.

5. Oxygen tank connected to isoflurane machine.

6. Isoflurane.

7. Carbon cartridge halogen filters connected to tubing to scavenge isoflurane.

8. Sterile petroleum jelly eye ointment (Fisher Scientific, Cat# NC0138063).

9. Extra mouse cage for anesthesia recovery.

10. Balance with 0.01 g accuracy and maximum capacity of at least 200 g.

3 Methods

All animal procedures should be reviewed and approved by your Institutional Animal Care and Use Committee.

Prior to Loading Experiment:

3.1 Loading Parameter Selection

1. Select peak or maximum compressive load. Peak or maximum load is the load level that will be reached repeatedly during the cyclic loading. This load can vary depending on age, sex, strain, and genotype. To determine this load level, in vivo strain gauging at the tibial midshaft should be performed (*see* Subheading 3.2 below). By determining tibial bone stiffness at the midshaft, the load to produce a desired strain at the tibial midshaft can be chosen.

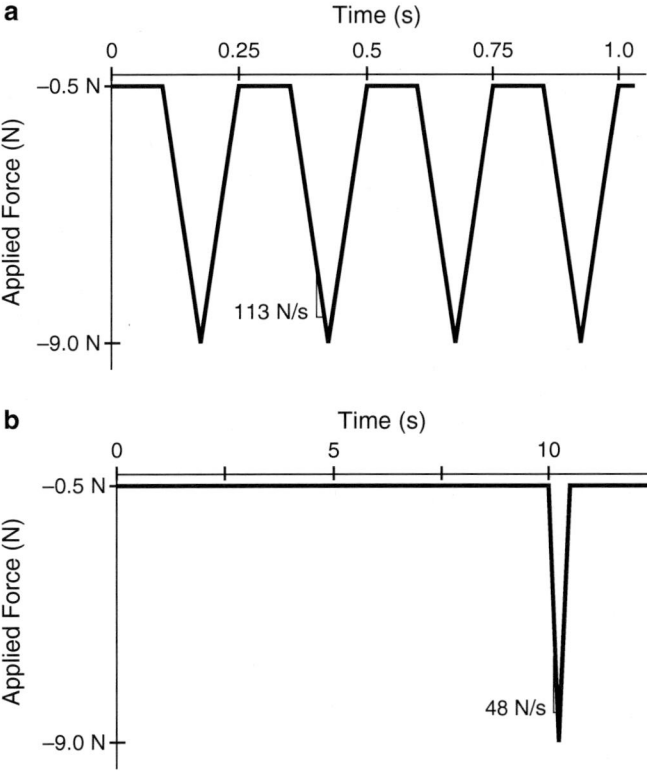

Fig. 1 Common in vivo axial tibial loading triangular waveforms for mice with 9.0 N peak compressive load. (**a**) This waveform is usually run five times per week, 1,200 cycles per day at a rate of 4 Hz, with a 0.1-s dwell period, and 113 N/s loading rate [8]. (**b**) This waveform is run three times per week, 60 cycles per day at a rate of 0.1 Hz, with a 10.0-s dwell period and a 48 N/s loading rate [9]

2. Select pre-load value. The magnitude of the compressive pre-load should be a small percentage of the maximum or peak load. For example, −0.5 N is an appropriate pre-load for a −9.0 N compressive peak load (*see* **Note 3**).

3. Select frequency, loading rate, dwell time, and number of cycles for the loading waveform. Triangle waves are generally used because the load is applied at a constant strain rate. For a sinusoidal wave, the loading rate varies throughout the cycle. One commonly used in vivo compressive loading protocol for the mouse consists of 1,200 cycles per day at 4 Hz, with a load-unload ramp of 0.15 and 0.1-s dwell time (Fig. 1) [8]. Another common protocol applies 60 cycles per day at 2 Hz, with a load-unload ramp of 0.15 and 10-s dwell time [9] (*see* **Note 4**).

4. Select pause insertion duration. Bone formation is stimulated by inserting pauses in between load cycles, rather than continuous cyclic loading [21]. In axial tibial loading of mice, rest insertions

have been short (0.1 s) or long (10.0 s) [8, 9]. As described in **step 3** pauses also can be used to achieve the desired loading rate and frequency.

5. Select loading duration. A range of loading durations have been used. Loading three or five times per week is most common [8, 9]. The duration of loading experiments can last from 1 day to 6 weeks and will depend on the research question and outcome measurements. Shorter time frames are often used when the primary outcome measures are skeletal gene expression changes after mechanical loading. Longer time frames are often used to detect changes in bone morphology, geometry, and cellular activity.

3.2 Determining In Vivo Stiffness Using Strain Gauges

Strain gauges are electrical conductors that change resistance when deformed. By rigidly attaching a gauge to the surface of the tibia, the deformation caused by loading can be measured. Stiffness is then calculated as the applied load per deformation. In practice, the goal is to determine the load required to achieve a desired strain level on the bone surface. For a stiff bone, this load is higher than for a more compliant bone.

3.2.1 Strain Gauge Preparation (Fig. 2)

1. Trim the gauge of unnecessary material. Place gauge on an index card and view using a dissecting microscope. Using a scalpel, remove excess material by cutting just within alignment markings; be careful not to disturb strain-sensitive grid. Use rocking motions, not shearing motions, to trim. Once trimmed, secure and protect grid with scotch tape while leaving terminals exposed.

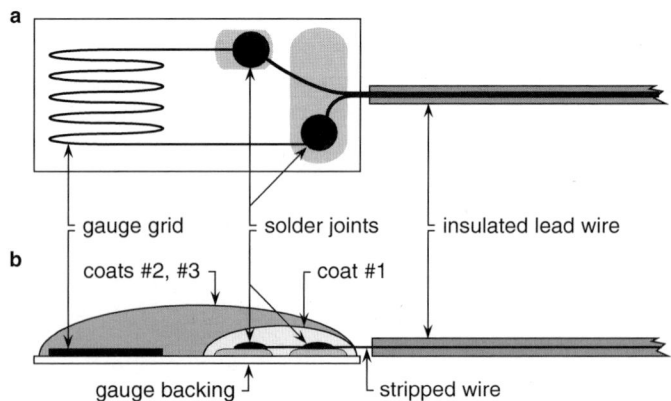

Fig. 2 Trimmed strain gauge assembly. (**a**) Top view of strain gauge preparation. (**b**) Side-view schematic of strain gauge preparation. The first coat is applied only to the soldering joint and should not touch the gauge grid. The second and third coats are applied to the entire gauge top surface. Stripped wire should not be exposed and can be covered by the coats

2. Prepare lead wires. Trim two wires to 17 cm in length and strip approximately 0.5 cm of insulation from one end of each wire. Dip these ends in solder flux and touch the soldering iron to each wire.

3. Prepare gauge terminals. Apply a minimal amount of solder primer to the end of each wire, and then use soldering iron to add tin. Use the dissecting microscope, and be careful to ensure that the added tin is contained within each terminal to prevent a short circuit.

4. Solder lead wires onto gauge terminals using the stripped and tinned ends.

5. Remove tape, and clean gauge with isopropyl alcohol.

6. Bend the gauge wires into an S shape so that the gauge is slanted with the grid section at the highest point.

7. Apply insulating coats (*see* **Note 5**).

(A) Mix up M-coat AE in a weigh boat 30 min before application to gauge leads. Mix a dime-sized amount of resin and two medicine drops of catalyst. After 30 min, apply only to the gauge terminals by dabbing small amounts of resin to the leads by touching with a wooden applicator stick. Make sure that the resin does not touch the grid. Let the resin catalyze overnight at room temperature.

(B) The following day, apply M-coat D (white, store in refrigerator) with the supplied brush to the entire upper surface of the gauge. Cure overnight at room temperature, or at room temperature for 15 min and then in an oven for 1 h at 65 °C (*see* **Note 6**).

8. The following day, apply M-coat A (clear, stored in refrigerator) to the entire top surface of the gauge using a wooden applicator stick by dab touching. Cure for 4–5 days at room temperature before applying the strain gauges to the bone (*see* **Note 7**).

9. Attach a plug to the wire ends. First apply flux to both the wire tips and the plug leads. Then, apply solder to the plug leads. Last, place the wires on top of the solder-covered plugs and heat with the soldering iron until bonded.

10. Coat plug/wire connections with epoxy.

11. Check the resistance of the gauge. Using a digital multimeter, touch the leads of the device to the ends of the plug. The strain gauge should read 120.0Ω, but an acceptable range is 118.5–121.5Ω.

3.2.2 In Vivo Load-Strain Calibration

1. Prepare a working area in a fume hood or biosafety cabinet.

2. Anesthetize the mouse using isoflurane (2.5 % in 1 L/min O_2). This procedure applies strain gauges as a non-survival surgery,

and so the mouse is anesthetized throughout the surgery and data collection and then euthanized.

3. Shave the mouse limb. Fur must be removed at the site of strain gauge application, which is the medial aspect of the hindlimb of interest.

4. Measure the length of the tibia from ankle to knee using calipers. Use the result to approximate the tibial midshaft and mark this location on the skin using a felt-tipped pen.

5. Incise the hindlimb to expose tibia. This exposure is most easily accomplished using scissors. First, make an opening where the midshaft was approximated. Then, using blunt dissection techniques separate skin from underlying muscle working proximally toward the knee and distally toward the ankle. The incision should be as small as possible, but will usually span from just proximal to the ankle joint to just distal to the knee joint. Keep in mind that the knee and ankle will be contact points when load is applied; therefore skin in these areas should remain intact.

6. Retract muscle and skin from implantation site. Use blunt dissection techniques to expose the periosteal surface of the tibia.

7. Prepare the tibial surface for adhesion. Gently scrape the bone with a periosteal elevator to remove the periosteum and debris. Degrease the bone using a cotton swab saturated with methyl ethyl ketone or chloroform.

8. Prepare strain gauge for adhesion. Using a cotton swab saturated with methyl ethyl ketone, degrease the gauge carefully using minimal pressure. Then, grasp the wires with jeweler's forceps just above the gauge.

9. Apply a very small drop of cyanoacrylate adhesive to the back of the gauge and immediately adhere the gauge to the midshaft of the tibia, being sure to align it with the long axis of the diaphysis (Fig. 3). Adhering the gauge works best when another laboratory member is firmly holding the tibia in place. Apply gentle pressure for 1 min to ensure secure attachment (*see* **Note 8**).

10. Examine the gauge attachment. The grid should be located at the midshaft of the tibia, aligned with the longitudinal axis of the tibia, and not be medial or lateral or rotated.

11. Calibrate the strain gauge. Open Labview or similar data acquisition software. Insert the gauge lead wires into strain conditioner or similar to complete the Wheatstone bridge quarter-bridge. Calibrate the gauge to zero while the mouse lies in a dorsal recumbent position. If calibration fails, a new gauge must be prepared and attached. To do so, the bone must be re-cleaned and the **steps 7–11** repeated.

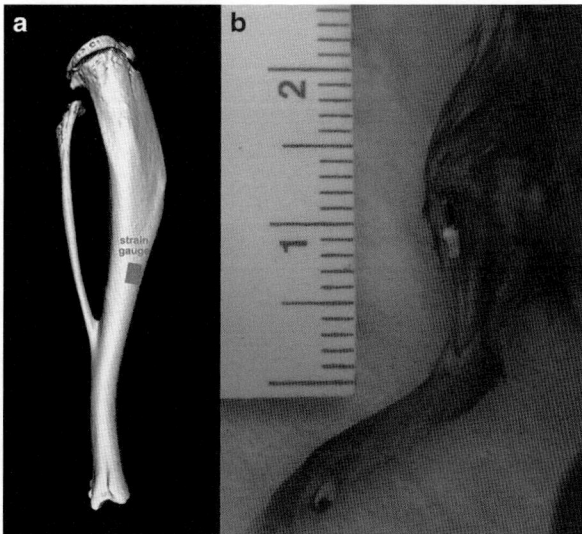

Fig. 3 Proper strain gauge placement at the tibial midshaft. (**a**) Schematic showing strain gauge positioned at the middiaphysis of tibia. (**b**) Photograph of surgically implanted gauge attached to surface of mouse tibia

12. Apply compressive load. Place animal in the loading device actuator and apply a voltage corresponding to approximately a 2 N load (*see* **Note 9**). Ascertain the viability of the attached gauge by determining if the results resemble accurate strain patterns. Apply mechanical loads for varying voltages to produce peak compressive loads from approximately 2.0 to 10.0 N (*see* **Note 10**).

13. Once all data have been collected, cut off the wires very close to the gauge, but keep the gauge attached to the bone. The tibia should be imaged using micro-computed tomography to determine if gauge placement was accurate. Gauge positioning is very important to ensure that results are comparable across different animals and ages.

14. Properly euthanize mouse once strain gauge data have been obtained for both limbs.

15. From stiffness data of all animals in a group, calculate the load needed to apply a specific strain to the tibial midshaft. The physiologic range of bone strain across multiple vertebrate species during normal activity is 1,000–1,500 μe in compression [22].

16. If desired, the strain data measured at the gauge location can be combined with a finite element analysis to determine the peak strain within the cortical cross section [9, 23]. The strains at the gauge location are generally not the maximum strains for the cortex. This analysis requires solving for the tibial strains using a computational model of the mouse tibia at the section of gauge attachment.

**3.3 In Vivo Axial
Tibial Loading
Experimental Methods**

*3.3.1 Setup
and Preparation for In Vivo
Axial Tibial Loading*

1. Connect and power on all electronic signal conditioning components, including the loading device.

2. Open LabView loading program and insert proper loading parameters.

3. Zero the load cell. Check load offset by reading load when load cell is resting without any item positioned in the loading fixtures. Depending on your loading system, either enter the load offset in Newtons if an offset is entered directly or select the option to zero the load cell. The load from load cell should now read 0.0 N (*see* **Note 11**).

4. Position a wooden rod in the loading device. Adjust and lock the horizontal position such that the rod is snug between the actuator and the load cell, but not so tight that the load cell is loaded beyond –1.0 N.

5. Open and appropriately name the data file.

6. Run practice loading session with rod to check components and confirm that the loading setup is working correctly and has no unforeseen issues.

*3.3.2 Application
of In Vivo Axial Tibial
Loading*

1. While rod is being loaded, turn on oxygen tank and isoflurane machine. Set oxygen flow to 1 L/min and isoflurane flow to 2 %, or whatever levels have been established in your protocol and approved by your Institutional Animal Care and Use Committee.

2. Place first mouse to be loaded into anesthesia chamber (Mouse A).

3. When Mouse A is asleep, remove Mouse A from chamber and apply eye ointment to each eye to maintain hydration during anesthesia, loading, and recovery.

4. When test of wooden rod completes, promptly loosen fixtures and remove the rod.

5. Immediately check the load cell offset and adjust offset value if necessary so that the resting load cell reads 0.0 N.

6. Remove Mouse A from the anesthesia chamber and place nose cone over nose.

7. Position Mouse A in the loading device, and lock the device so that the left tibia is snug. The left knee should be snug at the load cell cup and foot snug at the actuator (Fig. 4). Once tibia is positioned and the device adjusted and locked, load cell should not read below –1.0 N before loading begins or too much compressive pre-load is applied to the tibia (*see* **Note 12**).

8. Open a new data file and name the file appropriately to identify experiment, mouse, and date.

9. Begin the loading program when Mouse A's breathing is slowed.

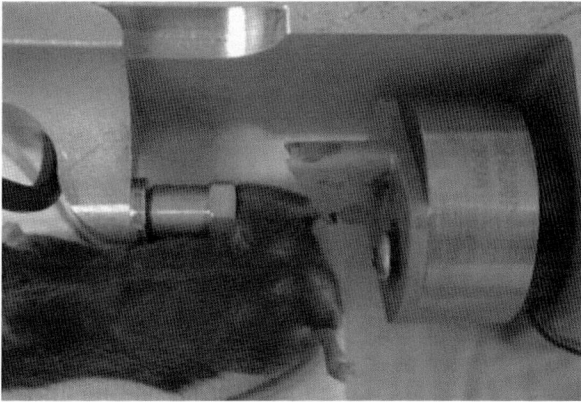

Fig. 4 Mouse situated in loading device, ready for in vivo axial loading to be applied to the left tibia

10. Monitor Mouse A during loading to check for continued slow breathing and unconsciousness (*see* **Note 13**).

11. Monitor the load cell and voltage outputs during the loading program (*see* **Note 14**).

12. When 2–3 min remains in the loading program, place the next mouse (Mouse B) into the isoflurane chamber (*see* **Note 15**).

13. When Mouse B is asleep, remove Mouse B from chamber and apply eye ointment to each eye to maintain hydration during anesthesia, loading, and recovery.

14. Once loading program finishes, promptly unlock the loading device, remove Mouse A, and place on balance.

15. Check the load cell offset and adjust offset value if necessary so that the resting load cell reads 0.0 N.

16. Record Mouse A body mass and place the animal into anesthesia recovery cage. Use one recovery cage per cage of mice. Once all mice from a single cage have been loaded, make sure that all mice are awake and moving around before returning the animals to their original cage.

17. Position Mouse B into loading device, and adjust and lock the device so that left tibia is snug.

18. Repeat **steps 7–17** for each subsequent mouse until all mice are loaded (Mouse B becomes Mouse A, next mouse becomes Mouse B, etc.).

19. If a mouse loses >10 % body mass over the course of an experiment, then wet food should be placed in the cage containing that mouse. If a mouse loses 20 % body mass, that mouse should no longer be used for the experiment and should be appropriately euthanized.

20. Repeat procedure for each day that mice are to be loaded. Always load the same tibia for each mouse.

3.3.3 Cleanup

1. Once final mouse is in recovery cage, turn off isoflurane and oxygen.
2. Close loading program software.
3. Turn off all electronic components.

3.4 Potential Outcome Measures

1. Cortical and cancellous morphology by micro-computed tomography.
2. Gene expression by qRT-PCR.
3. Dynamic histomorphometry using fluorochrome labeling.
4. Protein localization by immunohistochemistry.
5. Serum hormone assays by ELISA.
6. Many others.

4 Notes

1. The loads can be applied using a load-controlled mechanical testing system, such as the Bose Enduratec system or similar, or using a custom loading device with load cell and associated electronics signal conditioning hardware (National Instruments) and control software (Labview). When using a mechanical testing system, the loading waveform needs to be programmed within the software interface. Portable systems allow loading to be performed in the animal facility; tabletop machines require transportation of the animals to the laboratory. Custom loading devices are portable and allow loading in the animal facility. The Labview software can be customized as desired.
2. The practice rod does not have to be made of wood or be exactly 17 mm in length. Wooden handles removed from long cotton swabs work well because they approximate the length of a mouse tibia and are less stiff than metal.
3. A pre-load is required so that the actuator does not lift off at the beginning of loading or during the dwell phase of the cyclic loading.
4. Several loading waveform parameters are coupled. For example, loading rate and frequency are related. However, if the loading rate results in a higher frequency than desired, a dwell period may be included to achieve the desired frequency.
5. Insulating coats are applied to solidify solder bonds and to waterproof the gauge.
6. Toluene may be added to thin M-coat D as necessary.
7. Xylene may be added to thin M-coat A as necessary.
8. Attaching the strain gauge to bone in vivo is a difficult step, and practice runs are recommended.

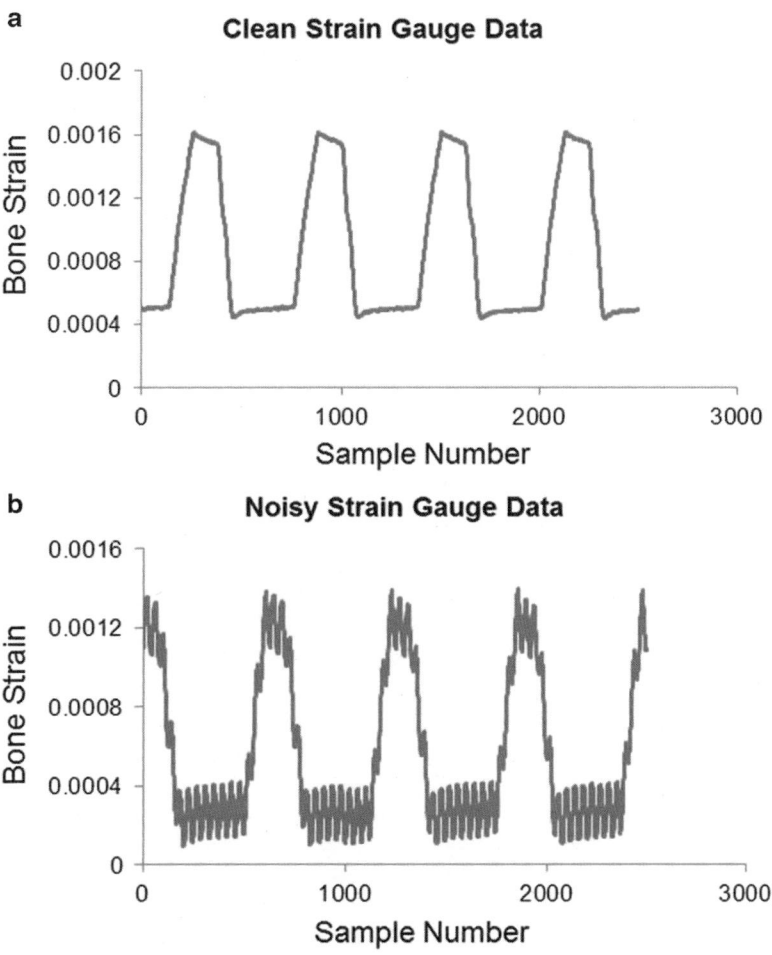

Fig. 5 Sample strain gauge data. (**a**) Clean data with clear values, indicating proper gauge attachment. (**b**) Data with high-frequency noise evident likely because the gauge is poorly attached or may be aligned off-axis. A new gauge should be used

9. This voltage should be determined prior to beginning strain gauge surgery. By loading a wooden rod in the loading device, the voltage corresponding to 2, 4, 6, 8, 10, and 12 N can be determined. These values can then be applied once the strain gauge is applied to the anesthetized mouse.

10. During strain gauging, several items must be monitored: (1) Noise in data: If the gauge is not attached properly or is mis-aligned, the data will be very noisy (Fig. 5). Occasionally this noise will decrease at higher voltages. If the noise does not disappear, then a new gauge needs to be attached and data collection must be repeated. (2) Strain levels: During loading, the bone strain should be approximated by determining the difference between the peak and valley of the strain readout. If the applied strain exceeds 2,000 µe as the voltage increases,

then the higher voltages should be excluded for this particular mouse/strain/limb. At very high strain levels, the bone could fracture. (3) Mouse status: Be sure that the mouse is in deep anesthesia and that its nose remains in the nose cone at all times.

11. The offset load for the load cell should stay relatively constant throughout the day and throughout the entire experiment. If large changes are noted, the load cell should be recalibrated or replaced. The offset load value should also be relatively low compared to the peak load applied to the tibia, at least <10 % but ideally <5 %.

12. The tibia is positioned horizontally in our loading device at Cornell, and so the mouse will be positioned on its back. If the tibia is positioned vertically, the mouse will be positioned differently.

13. If the mouse's breathing becomes rapid, quickly increase the isoflurane to 2.5–3 % for a period of about 20 s. For the next mouse, be sure to wait longer for slower breathing before beginning the loading program.

14. Both the voltage input and load output should be steady cyclic wave patterns. Make sure that peak load is being reached consistently. If using Labview and input and/or output are jumpy, Hardware Configuration PID settings may need to be altered. If load cell is not reading, immediately stop program and check that all wires are connected.

15. This time to start anesthesia may vary depending on how quickly anesthesia takes effect on mice and will differ by age, sex, and genotype.

Acknowledgments

We would like to acknowledge our funding sources: NIH R01-AG028664 (MCHM), R01-AR53237 (AGR) and I01-BX001478 (AGR), and NSF GRFP (KMM). We would also like to thank the following individuals who have been involved in the development of these methods: Dr. J. Christopher Fritton, Dr. Maureen E. Lynch, and Dr. Russell P. Main.

References

1. Turner CH, Akhter MP, Raab DM et al (1991) A noninvasive, in vivo model for studying strain adaptive bone modeling. Bone 12: 73–79

2. Lee KC, Maxwell A, Lanyon LE (2002) Validation of a technique for studying functional adaptation of the mouse ulna in response to mechanical loading. Bone 31:407–412

3. Fritton JC, Myers ER, Wright TM et al (2005) Loading induces site-specific increases in mineral content assessed by microcomputed tomography of the mouse tibia. Bone 36:1030–1038

4. Wallace JM, Rajachar RM, Allen MR et al (2007) Exercise-induced changes in the cortical bone of growing mice are bone- and gender-specific. Bone 40:1120–1127

5. Prisby RD, Lafage-Proust MH, Malaval L et al (2008) Effects of whole body vibration on the skeleton and other organ systems in man and animal models: What we know and what we need to know. Ageing Res Rev 7:319–329

6. Iwamoto J, Takeda T, Sato Y (2005) Effect of treadmill exercise on bone mass in female rats. Exp Anim 54:1–6

7. De Souza RL, Matsuura M, Eckstein F et al (2005) Non-invasive axial loading of mouse tibiae increases cortical bone formation and modifies trabecular organization: a new model to study cortical and cancellous compartments in a single loaded element. Bone 37:810–818

8. Lynch ME, Main RP, Xu Q et al (2010) Cancellous bone adaptation to tibial compression is not sex dependent in growing mice. J Appl Physiol 109:685–691

9. Brodt MD, Silva MJ (2010) Aged mice have enhanced endocortical response and normal periosteal response compared with young-adult mice following 1 week of axial tibial compression. J Bone Miner Res 25:2006–2015

10. Sheng MH, Baylink DJ, Beamer WG et al (1999) Histomorphometric studies show that bone formation and bone mineral apposition rates are greater in C3H/HeJ (high-density) than C57BL/6J (low-density) mice during growth. Bone 25:421–429

11. Klein RF, Shea M, Gunness ME et al (2001) Phenotypic characterization of mice bred for high and low peak bone mass. J Bone Miner Res 16:63–71

12. Wergedal JE, Sheng MH, Ackert-Bicknell CL et al (2005) Genetic variation in femur extrinsic strength in 29 different inbred strains of mice is dependent on variations in femur cross-sectional geometry and bone density. Bone 36:11–22

13. Sabsovich I, Clark JD, Liao G et al (2008) Bone microstructure and its associated genetic variability in 12 inbred mouse strains: microCT study and in silico genome scan. Bone 42:439–451

14. Beamer WG, Donahue LR, Rosen CJ et al (1996) Genetic variability in adult bone density among inbred strains of mice. Bone 18:397–403

15. Robling AG, Turner CH (2002) Mechanotransduction in bone: genetic effects on mechanosensitivity in mice. Bone 31:562–569

16. Saxon LK, Robling AG, Castillo AB et al (2007) The skeletal responsiveness to mechanical loading is enhanced in mice with a null mutation in estrogen receptor-beta. Am J Physiol Endocrinol Metab 293:484–491

17. Nielsen RH, Christiansen C, Stolina M et al (2008) Oestrogen exhibits type II collagen protective effects and attenuates collagen-induced arthritis in rats. Clin Exp Immunol 152:21–27

18. Glatt V, Canalis E, Stadmeyer L et al (2007) Age-related changes in trabecular architecture differ in female and male C57BL/6J mice. J Bone Miner Res 22:1197–1207

19. Sample SJ, Collins RJ, Wilson AP et al (2010) Systemic effects of ulna loading in male rats during functional adaptation. J Bone Miner Res 25:2016–2028

20. Sugiyama T, Price JS, Lanyon LE (2010) Functional adaptation to mechanical loading in both cortical and cancellous bone is controlled locally and is confined to the loaded bones. Bone 46:314–321

21. Srinivasan S, Ausk BJ, Poliachik SL et al (2007) Rest-inserted loading rapidly amplifies the response of bone to small increases in strain and load cycles. J Appl Physiol 102:1945–1952

22. Rubin CT, Lanyon LE (1984) Dynamic strain similarity in vertebrates; an alternative to allometric limb bone scaling. J Theor Biol 107:321–327

23. Christiansen BA, Bayly PV, Silva MJ (2008) Constrained tibial vibration in mice: a method for studying the effects of vibrational loading of bone. J Biomech Eng 130:044502

Chapter 10

Four-Point Bending Protocols to Study the Effects of Dynamic Strain in Osteoblastic Cells In Vitro

Gabriel L. Galea and Joanna S. Price

Abstract

Strain engendered within bone tissue by mechanical loading of the skeleton is a major influence on the processes of bone modeling and remodeling and so a critical determinant of bone mass and architecture. The cells best placed to respond to strain in bone tissue are the resident osteocytes and osteoblasts. To address the mechanisms of strain-related responses in osteoblast-like cells, our group uses both in vivo and in vitro approaches, including a system of four-point bending of the substrate on which cells are cultured. A range of cell lines can be studied using this system but we routinely compare their responses to those in primary cultures of osteoblast-like cells derived from explants of mouse long bones. These cells show a range of well-characterized responses to physiological levels of strain, including increased proliferation, which in vivo is a feature of the osteogenic response.

Key words Mechanical loading, Bone, Strain, Mechanobiology, Four-point bending, Osteoblast

1 Introduction

When healthy, bones adapt their structure and material properties to withstand habitual levels of everyday loading without suffering fracture or the undue accumulation of micro-damage. To achieve this, bone mass and architecture are adjusted in relation to changes in their load-bearing environment through a feedback loop in which the activity of cells responsible for formation and resorption is influenced by the mechanical strains they experience. Harold Frost [1, 2] first used the term "the mechanostat" to liken this homeostatic loop to a household thermostat, although the simplicity of this analogy belies the complex nature of the biological processes by which bone cells sense, transduce, and respond appropriately to loading-engendered stimuli. To identify characteristics of the loading regime (peak strain, maximum strain rate, strain distribution, etc.) that influence bones' subsequent adaptive response [3], investigators have used a variety of animal models [4–7]. In recent years the mouse has become the preferred animal model

Jennifer J. Westendorf and Andre J. van Wijnen (eds.), *Osteoporosis and Osteoarthritis*, Methods in Molecular Biology, vol. 1226, DOI 10.1007/978-1-4939-1619-1_10, © Springer Science+Business Media New York 2015

because artificial loading of bones in genetically modified mice enables the role of specific genes and pathways to be investigated in vivo [8–10].

A limitation of in vivo models is that they are unsuitable for studying the cellular and molecular mechanisms. Thus, in vitro models are also required, even though they cannot replicate the complex interactions between resident bone cells that exist in vivo. Our lab and many others working in the bone mechanobiology field now use both in vivo and in vitro systems to investigate the mechanisms of the mechanostat with the aim of developing rational therapeutic strategies for treating bone disease.

For many years our group has studied the effects of mechanical strain in vitro with a four-point bending technique applied to plastic slides covered with cells. Advantages of in vitro four-point bending systems include the ability to engender physiological strains in a uniform distribution and uniaxial direction over the culture surface. Several slides (six in our system) can be strained simultaneously, providing technical repeats. Strains engendered in the cells' substrate can be quantified through strain gauging in order to validate the system. The peak strain magnitude normally applied in our experiments is 3,400 $\mu\varepsilon$ as similar magnitudes of strain have been measured on the cortex of a variety of bones subjected to physiological loading in vivo [11]. Strain "dose-response" studies show that this magnitude of strain triggers the greatest increase in osteoblast proliferation and estrogen receptor (ER) response element activity [12, 13]. Similar systems of substrate strain by four-point bending have been developed by other groups [14, 15] and commercially available substrate strain systems, including the Flexercell system, are also available [16–19].

A limitation of our four-point bending system is the requirement for a large number of cells to study specific experimental end points, e.g., protein quantification by western blotting or mRNA analysis quantitative PCR. Secondly, four-point bending engenders some turbulent fluid flow over the cells which cannot be quantified [20]. Since fluid flow is a natural consequence of bone loading in vivo and also influences bone cell behavior, many groups use systems designed to expose cells to pulsed fluid flow on the assumption that this is the natural primary strain-related stimulus for resident bone cells [21]. However, the limitation of using fluid flow as a mechanical stimulus is that the shear strains engendered are nonuniform and difficult to quantify due to the deformation of cellular processes [22].

Investigators use a variety of cell types in the model systems described above. Osteoblasts when entombed within the bone matrix terminally differentiate to form osteocytes, which are widely believed to coordinate (re)modeling in response to changes in loading in vivo. Because of their anatomical location and the fact that they do not divide, osteocytes have been challenging cells to study.

Historically, our group and others investigated the effects of substrate strain and fluid flow on primary cultures of osteocytes by extracting these cells from chick bones using the Mab 7.3 antibody [23]. Consistent responses to strain observed in these osteocytic cells include the release of nitric oxide, prostacyclin, and prostaglandin E2 [23]. Unfortunately, Mab 7.3 is no longer being produced and although alternative techniques to extract osteocyte-rich fractions from adult mouse bones are now available, they yield relatively small numbers of cells [24]. For this reason some of the most significant advances in our understanding of osteocyte mechanotransduction have been achieved by groups investigating the response of osteocytic cell lines, including Mlo-Y4 cells, to fluid flow shear stress [22, 25–27].

Unlike osteocytes, osteoblasts on bone surfaces are unlikely to be exposed to fluid flow as they are not located within a canalicular network. However, differentiated osteoblasts respond as rapidly as osteocytes to in vivo loading and do so in a strain-magnitude-related manner [28, 29]. Even marrow stromal cells, which are not well placed to detect strains within bone tissue, respond to substrate strain by increasing their activation of the canonical Wnt secondary messenger β-catenin which promotes their differentiation into osteoblasts [17–19]. Recent studies show that this stimulus promotes their differentiation along an osteoblastic rather than an adipogenic phenotype [17, 18].

To study osteoblasts' responses to strain, a large number of different cell lines are available, and several have been used by our group over the years and have played a role in identifying the complexity of strain-related signaling pathways (reviewed in [30, 31]). In response to strain, ROS 17/2.8 rat osteosarcoma cells proliferate, activate genomic estrogen response elements, increase phosphorylation of ERK and of the estrogen receptor ERα, and increase levels of active β-catenin [12, 20, 32, 33]. UMR-106 cells are a rat osteosarcoma cell line in which strain increases active β-catenin levels independently of LRP5 through a process involving insulin-like growth factor receptor signaling facilitated by ERα [34]. We used UMR-106 cells to study the mechanisms by which strain up-regulates the expression of the early response gene EGR2, which was identified using an in vivo microarray study [35, 36]. More recently, our group has begun to use Saos-2 human female osteosarcoma cells because of their physiological expression of the osteocytic product *Sost*/sclerostin [37–39]. When sub-confluent, Saos-2 cells proliferate following exposure to strain similarly to primary osteoblasts [38]. However, when over-confluent, Saos-2 cells increase their expression of *Sost* and downregulate *Sost* expression over a time course congruent with that observed following in vivo loading of rodent bones [37, 38].

Wherever practical, we aim to validate findings obtained using cell lines in primary osteoblast-like cells. Osteoblast-like cells can be readily obtained from serially digested neonatal rodent calvariae.

However, the flat bones of the calvarium are not load bearing and as such are of questionable relevance to studies investigating the mechanisms by which loading modifies the mass and architecture of long bones. In vivo, long bones and flat bones retain distinct gene signatures related to their embryological origin [40] and, in vitro, osteoblastic cells derived from the calvariae of rats show different responses to mechanical strain to cells explanted from the long bones of the same animals [41]; for example, long bone but not calvarium-derived osteoblastic cells show strain-related increases in the activity of the metabolizing enzyme G6PD [41].

To study long bone-derived osteoblasts' responses to strain, our group developed a method of explanting cells from the load-bearing cortices of adult mice. Cells explanted following our protocol express osteoblastic markers including alkaline phosphatase and osteocalcin, mineralize their matrix when treated with ascorbic acid and β-glycerol phosphate, and show a range of responses to physiological substrate strain in our system [38, 42, 43]. These responses include the release of prostaglandins and nitric oxide, nuclear accumulation of β-catenin, and up-regulating the expression of various target genes including EGR2, Cox2, and IL-11 following exposure to strain by four-point bending [33–35, 38, 42, 43]. Furthermore, a well-established response of osteoblast-like cells to strain in vitro is an increase in their proliferation [8, 38, 44]. Osteoblast proliferation is studied using various techniques including immunofluorescent staining for the proliferating cell marker Ki-67 directly on the slides on which cells are strained [38].

In this chapter we describe the methods required to study the effects of strain by four-point substrate bending on osteoblast proliferation. We first describe the methods required to strain gauge plastic slides in vitro. This is done to ensure a uniform distribution of substrate strain at the desired physiological peak strain magnitude. The method we use for explanting of cortical long bone-derived osteoblasts (CLBObs) will first be described, followed by the method used to investigate the effect of strain on their proliferation.

2   Materials

2.1   Quantification of Mechanical Strain In Vitro

1. Custom-made, sterile, tissue culture-coated, flexible plastic strips ("slides") on which cells are cultured for in vitro strain experiments are made to order by Nunc (USA). Generate these slides by cutting the bottoms of 4-well plates, producing slides of a standard size (7.5×2.5 cm) with tissue culture coating on one side (Fig. 1).

2. Strain gauges (EA-06-015DJ-120), gauge adhesive glue, and a standard calibration resistor (1 Ω, M.M B9744S102C) are

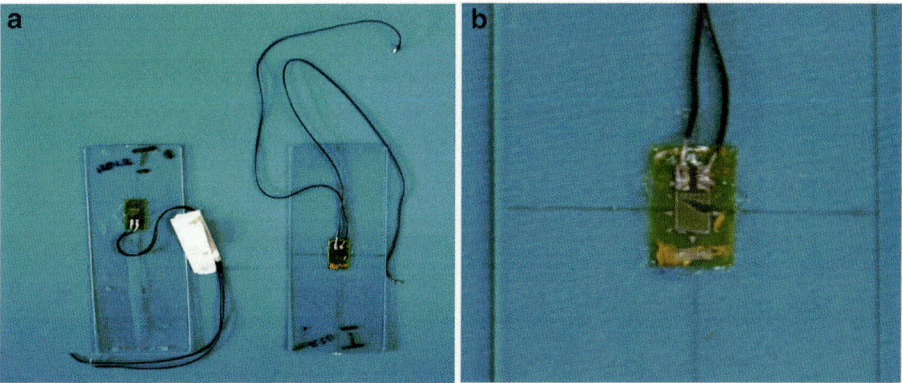

Fig. 1 Strain gauges bonded onto plastic cell culture slides are used to quantify strains generated by four-point bending. (**a**) Strain gauges are attached at different positions on each slide. (**b**) Magnified view of a strain gauge attached to the center of a slide

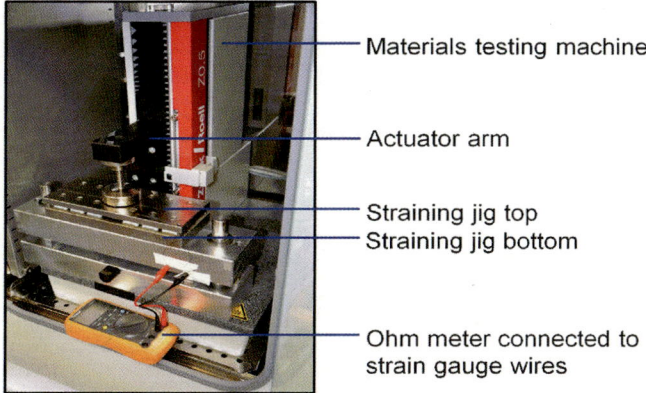

Materials testing machine

Actuator arm

Straining jig top
Straining jig bottom

Ohm meter connected to strain gauge wires

Fig. 2 The Zwick/Roëll materials testing machine used to generate strain in vitro. The materials testing machine is permanently housed inside a cell culture incubator kept at 37 °C. The various components are labeled

from Vishay Measurements Group (Basingstoke, UK). Strain gauges are designed such that a change in strain causes a linear change in their internal resistance.

3. Ohm meter (or resistance transducer connected to an oscilloscope which illustrates a visible trace representing changes in resistance measured by the transducer).

4. Zwick/Roëll upright materials testing machine (Zwick Testing Machines Ltd., Leominster, UK) (Fig. 2) housed permanently inside a standard cell culture incubator maintained at 37 °C and 5 % CO_2.

5. A mobile, sterile, stainless steel "straining jig" insert. This was designed by Professor Lennart Stromberg (Karolinska Institute, Sweden) and custom made at University College London.

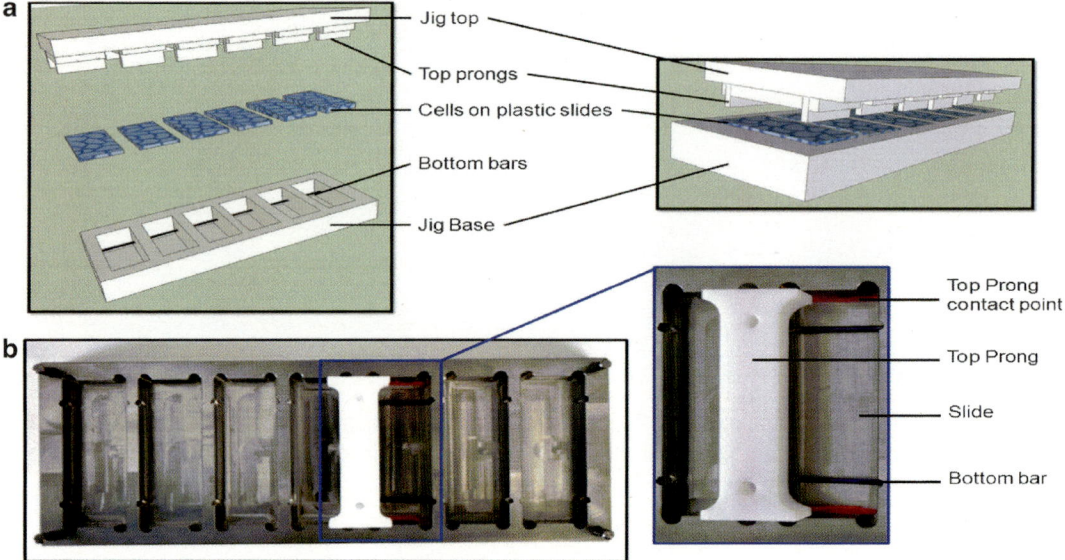

Fig. 3 Construction of the sterile straining jig insert. (**a**) Schematic representation of the straining jig insert in open and closed positions. (**b**) Straining jig bottom showing the wells with a slide in one well (magnified). The *white* prong is disconnected from the straining jig top to illustrate its approximate position relative to its contact points on the slide shown in *red*

This jig is composed of a base with wells into which the slides fit, and a removable top with plastic prongs that push down onto the slides as schematically represented in Fig. 3a. Springs at the four corners prevent the top exerting any force on the slides between strain cycles. Each of these wells contains a metal bar at each end (Fig. 3b) on top of which the slides rest.

2.2 Explanting Adult Mouse Long Bone-Derived Osteoblastic Cells

1. Long bones harvested from adult C57Bl/6 mice, typically 16–19 weeks of age.

2. Sterile dissection instruments to include fine scissors, fine and blunt forceps, rat-toothed forceps, size 11 and size 22 scalpel blades with handles.

3. 100× Antibiotic/antimycotic (AB/AM) solution diluted to 1× concentration in Dulbecco's phosphate-buffered saline (PBS + AB/AM).

4. 70 % ethanol solution in distilled water. This pot should be large enough to completely submerge a mouse (greater than 200 ml).

5. Complete medium: Phenol red-free Dulbecco's modified Eagle's medium (DMEM) with 10 % fetal bovine serum (FBS-Gold) (*see* **Note 1**).

6. Accutase (PAA).

2.3 Exposure of Osteoblast-Like Cells to Mechanical Strain In Vitro

1. Passage 1 osteoblast-like cells in suspension.
2. Plastic slides and the components of the straining system.
3. Complete medium described in Subheading 2.2, **item 5**.
4. Serum deprivation medium containing 2 % charcoal-dextran-stripped FBS Gold in DMEM.

3 Methods

3.1 Quantification of Mechanical Strain In Vitro

1. In vitro strain gauging is done to ensure that slides are exposed to the desired physiological strain of 3,400 $\mu\varepsilon$. Bond strain gauges onto slides with strain gauge adhesive glue by placing a small volume of glue directly onto the slide and then placing a strain gauge onto the glue using delicate forceps (*see* **Note 2**). Press the strain gauge down with the tips of the forceps at the edge of strain gauge until bonded to the slide surface. The strain gauge will have wires extending from its center through which resistance can be measured.

2. Determine the bonded strain gauge's baseline resistance by connecting the strain gauge wires to the Ohm meter (the connection mechanism will depend on the Ohm meter model used). Strain gauges are bonded and their resistance tested at different sites on the slide to ensure uniformity of strain distribution (Fig. 1a). Ohm meter accuracy is confirmed by using a standard resistor.

3. Using the materials testing machine's inbuilt controls, displace the jig top downwards to deform the slides as the top prongs are pushed down on either side of the bottom rods (Fig. 3b), resulting in uniform, uniaxial tensile strain in the upper surface of the slide and consequently a change in resistance in the strain gauge bonded to it (*see* **Note 3**). The maximum lever arm displacement used is that required to achieve a peak strain of 3,400 $\mu\varepsilon$ (*see* **Note 4**).

4. Expect a linear relationship between jig displacement and recorded strain magnitude and this relationship should be the same in all wells of the straining jig. Ensure the central application of force onto the staining jig top by the materials testing machine lever arm. Strain gauging results are shown in Fig. 4.

5. Use a waveform with rates on and off of 23,000 $\mu\varepsilon$/s, dwell times on and off of 0.7 s, and a peak strain of 3,400 $\mu\varepsilon$ with a frequency of approximately 0.6 Hz (*see* **Note 5**). To do this, program the desired dwell times, lever arm travel speed, and lever arm travel distances using the materials testing machine's inbuilt program (in the case of the Zwick/Roëll system a program wizard can be used to specify these steps). Repeat 600 times. Other waveforms and cycle numbers have been used in similar systems (for example [16]).

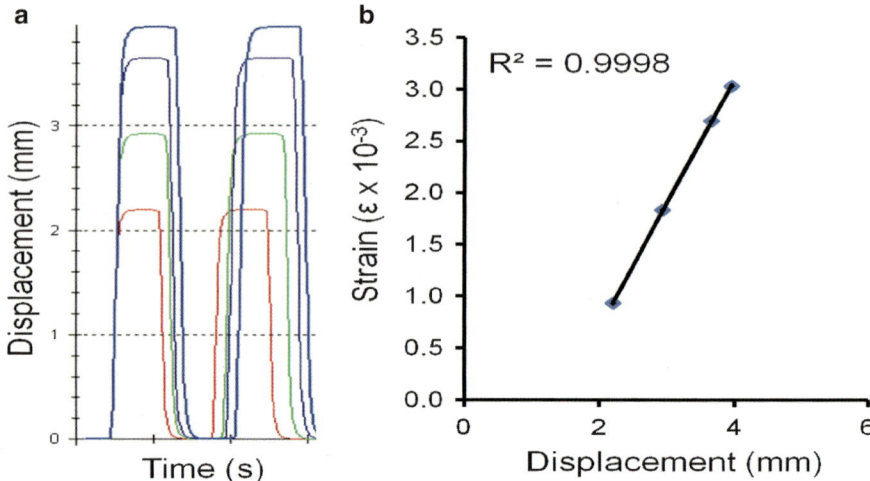

Fig. 4 Strain waveform and peak strains generated at different displacements. (**a**) The strain waveform is provided by the Zwick/Roëll materials testing analysis software at different pre-programmed peak displacements. (**b**) Representative strain gauging result illustrating the expected linear relationship between displacement of the materials testing machine lever arm (*see* Fig. 2) and the peak strain quantified as change in resistance

3.2 Explanting Mouse Long Bone-Derived Osteoblastic Cells

1. Sacrifice mice following Schedule 1 procedures, typically cervical dislocation, in accordance with the Animals (Scientific Procedures) Act of 1986. Mouse bodies are kept on ice until processed (*see* **Note 6**).

2. Submerge the entire mouse body in 70 % ethanol solution for approximately 1 min.

3. Make a circumferential incision in the skin around each hind limb at the level of the hip and peel back the skin using sterile rat-toothed forceps, preventing hair contamination. Excise the extrinsic muscles and disarticulate the femoral head from the acetabulum. Holding the limb by the foot, cut the tibia with scissors such that the limb falls in a fresh dish of sterile PBS+AB/AM. Keep limbs in this solution throughout the extraction.

4. Having disarticulated the hind limbs, similarly collect the forelimbs by making a circumferential incision around the limb, peeling back the skin, cutting through all extrinsic muscles, and then cutting just below the manus (*see* **Note 7**).

5. Section the limbs at each joint. To isolate cortical regions, cut the epiphyses and dissect away the surrounding muscles from the diaphyses using fine forceps and a size 11 scalpel blade. Take care to prevent excessively scraping the periosteum, but make the removal of contaminating muscle cells and fibroblasts a priority (*see* **Note 8**).

6. Remove marrow cells by sectioning the bones longitudinally with a size 11 scalpel blade, allowing easy access to the medullary cavity, and washing thoroughly by pipetting PBS + AB/AM until the bones appear white. Remove all the PBS and add fresh PBS + AB/AM to cover the bone fragments.

7. Section bone fragments with a size 22 scalpel into approximately 2 mm³ pieces and wash the pieces 2–3 times with fresh PBS + AB/AM. Section the remaining fragments further into the smallest possible pieces and transfer the resulting bone powder directly into a T75 flask containing 14 ml of complete medium.

8. Leave the resulting bone chips undisturbed for 1 week, following which cells are clearly visible growing directly out of the chips. Change half the medium on the CLBObs three times a week until nearly confluent, which is typically 3 weeks later when bones from a single mouse are explanted into a T75 flask.

9. To subculture CLBObs add accutase (7 ml/T75 flask, *see* **Note 9**) and incubate for 5 min at 37 °C. Pellet cells by centrifugation at 1,500 RPM (320×*g*) for 5 min at 4 °C. Always use passage CLBObs at passage 1 for experiments as described in Subheading 3.3.

3.3 Exposure of Cells to Mechanical Strain In Vitro

The procedure described here is that used to determine proliferation of CLBObs as previously described [38].

1. Place slides inside 4-well dishes or standard 120 mm cell culture dishes (up to five per dish, *see* **Note 10**).

2. Use cells from Subheading 3.2, **step 9**, to seed 100,000 CLBObs onto each slide in 0.5 ml complete medium (*see* **Note 11**). Spread this aliquot evenly over the surface of the slide using non-hydrophobic cell scrapers leaving an approximately 0.5 cm margin around the edges. Carefully carry the slides inside their dishes to a standard cell culture incubator at 37 °C, 5 % CO_2, 95 % humidity.

3. Allow the CLBObs to adhere to the slides overnight. The next day, add 5 ml of complete medium to each slide (*see* **Note 12**).

4. Following a further 24 h of culture in complete medium (48 h since seeding), completely replace medium with 10 ml of serum deprivation medium and incubate CLBObs overnight. This enhances the mitogenic effects of strain.

5. The following morning, pre-warm the sterilized straining jig to 37 °C and transfer slides to be strained into the jig wells. Place the jig in the Zwick/Roëll materials testing machine as illustrated in Fig. 3. Take control, static slides not subjected to strain in and out of the incubators with the strained slides.

6. Transfer the strained cells from the straining jig back into their dishes together with the medium they were strained in. Always keep the cells in the medium they were strained in for the remainder of the experiment. Fix or harvest cells from the slides as required (*see* **Notes 13–15**).

7. Between straining different groups, wash the jig with warm PBS.

4   Notes

1. Phenol red is avoided throughout, because this compound is a phytoestrogen and estrogen receptor signaling is an important component of osteoblastic cells' responses to strain [38, 43, 44]. The fetal bovine serum used is FBS Gold purchased from PAA (Yeovil, UK). Each lot is batch tested by confirming the formation of mineralized nodules and strain-related increases in proliferation of long bone osteoblastic cells.

2. Slightly scraping the surface of the slide with a scalpel blade facilitates gauge attachment. Strain gauging must be performed for each batch of slides. We normally bulk order a large batch (>10,000) slides in sterile packets of 10. When stored for a prolonged period of time the displacement:strain relationship in these slides can drift and repeated strain gauging is required.

3. Materials testing machines can either be set to apply a predefined force or achieve a predetermined displacement. We always use the displacement mode as this is the same irrespective of the number of slides being strained. Even in displacement mode, the materials testing machine applies a force through a load cell, which measures force and cuts out as a safety feature if its maximum load is exceeded. Compressing the jig springs and deforming the slides at the required strain rates easily exceed 20 N, so a large load cell is required.

4. In our experience, exposing the slides we use to more than ~4,000 $\mu\varepsilon$ risks damaging them. The 3,400 $\mu\varepsilon$ in vitro strain magnitude has been the "standard" used by our lab for many years [8, 33–35, 38, 42–44] and similar strains have been recorded on the surface of bones subjected to physiological osteogenic loading in vivo [45].

5. In our hands, the Zwick/Roëll upright materials testing machine delivers the desired strain waveform at a maximum frequency of approximately 0.6 Hz. Other waveforms and cycle numbers have been used in similar systems (for example [16]).

6. On occasion, mouse bodies have been shipped to us on wet ice overnight with no loss of viable cell yield.

7. We often collect the hind limbs for processing by different techniques and only explant CLBObs from the forelimb long bones. Forelimb bone chips from four to five mice are typically pooled into one T75 flask.

8. In practice, it is often necessary to scrape the surface of the bone with a size 11 scalpel blade to ensure that all muscle and loose connective tissue is removed. This does not prevent osteoblastic cells growing out of the bones. Sectioning through tuberosities, particularly the deltoid tuberosity in the humerus, greatly facilitates muscle removal.

9. Although standard trypsin/EDTA is used to subculture cell lines, accutase is used to subculture primary osteoblastic cells. Accutase is claimed by the manufacturer to contain a self-denaturing enzyme, which is less likely to cause damage to the cells.

10. Each well of 4-well dishes must be large enough to contain 10 ml of serum deprivation medium. Placing a drop of complete medium under each slide prevents movement in subsequent steps.

11. Seeding cells in 0.5 ml of medium causes the medium to stretch out over the surface of the slide. Larger volumes of medium form a dome over the center of the slide, causing a greater proportion of cells to settle in the center. However, up to 1 ml of medium may be required when very large numbers of cells must be seeded on each slide (e.g., 400,000 Saos-2 cells per slide when investigating *Sost* regulation as previously described [37, 38]).

12. When flooding slides, extreme care must be taken to ensure that the entire surface area of the slide is covered as otherwise the slide tends to float upwards such that the top may desiccate. It is also essential to ensure that no air bubbles form under the slides as these can cause the slide to float, desiccating the top surface on which cells are seeded.

13. To harvest cell lysates at the desired time points following strain, slides are fist washed in ice-cold PBS and kept in PBS on ice. Each slide is wedged firmly inside a 50 ml centrifuge tube and the required lysis buffer is added to the surface on which cells are adhered. The lysis buffer is spread with a cell scraper and the tube is then centrifuged with the slide inside it at 800 RPM for 5 min at 4 °C.

14. To fix cells for cytological processing, the slides are first washed in ice-cold PBS and then fixed as required.

15. One benefit of straining cells on slides, rather than flexible membranes, is that slides can be directly processed for immunocytochemistry and immunofluorescence. Immunofluorescence can be used to detect various proteins on plastic slides including

the Ki-67 proliferating cell marker as previously described [38]. Because plastic produces autofluorescence in the green spectrum, in our experience blue and red fluorochromes produce clearer immunofluorescent images by conventional fluorescent microscopy. If a green fluorochrome is required, Alexa 488 appears to produce clearer images than the commonly used FITC dye.

Acknowledgements

Much of the work described here was funded by the Wellcome Trust (to J.S.P.) and a Veterinary Intercalated Training Fellowship also from the Wellcome Trust (to G.L.G.).

References

1. Frost HM (1987) Bone "mass" and the "mechanostat": a proposal. Anat Rec 219:1–9

2. Frost HM (2003) Bone's mechanostat: a 2003 update. Anat Rec A Discov Mol Cell Evol Biol 275:1081–1101

3. Ehrlich PJ, Lanyon LE (2002) Mechanical strain and bone cell function: a review. Osteoporos Int 13:688–700

4. Rubin CT, Lanyon LE (1984) Regulation of bone formation by applied dynamic loads. J Bone Joint Surg Am 66:397–402

5. Turner CH, Akhter MP, Raab DM et al (1991) A noninvasive, in vivo model for studying strain adaptive bone modeling. Bone 12:73–79

6. Chambers TJ, Evans M, Gardner TN et al (1993) Induction of bone formation in rat tail vertebrae by mechanical loading. Bone Miner 20:167–178

7. Lee KC, Maxwell A, Lanyon LE (2002) Validation of a technique for studying functional adaptation of the mouse ulna in response to mechanical loading. Bone 31:407–412

8. Lee K, Jessop H, Suswillo R et al (2003) Endocrinology: bone adaptation requires oestrogen receptor-alpha. Nature 424(6947):389

9. Sawakami K, Robling AG, Ai M et al (2006) The Wnt co-receptor LRP5 is essential for skeletal mechanotransduction but not for the anabolic bone response to parathyroid hormone treatment. J Biol Chem 18:23698–23711

10. Trussel A, Muller R, Webster D et al (2012) Toward mechanical systems biology in bone. Ann Biomed Eng 40:2475–2487

11. Moustafa A, Sugiyama T, Prasad J et al (2012) Mechanical loading-related changes in osteocyte sclerostin expression in mice are more closely associated with the subsequent osteogenic response than the peak strains engendered. Osteoporos Int 23:1225–1234

12. Zaman G, Cheng MZ, Jessop HL et al (2000) Mechanical strain activates estrogen response elements in bone cells. Bone 27:233–239

13. Javaheri B, Sunters A, Zaman G et al (2012) Lrp5 is not required for the proliferative response of osteoblasts to strain but regulates proliferation and apoptosis in a cell autonomous manner. PLoS One 7:e35726

14. Xu T, Yang K, You H et al (2013) Regulation of PTHrP expression by cyclic mechanical strain in postnatal growth plate chondrocytes. Bone 56:304–311

15. Cai X, Zhang Y, Yang X et al (2011) Uniaxial cyclic tensile stretch inhibits osteogenic and odontogenic differentiation of human dental pulp stem cells. J Tissue Eng Regen Med 5:347–353

16. Aguirre JI, Plotkin LI, Gortazar AR et al (2007) A novel ligand-independent function of the estrogen receptor is essential for osteocyte and osteoblast mechanotransduction. J Biol Chem 282:25501–25508

17. Sen B, Xie Z, Case N et al (2008) Mechanical strain inhibits adipogenesis in mesenchymal stem cells by stimulating a durable beta-catenin signal. Endocrinology 149:6065–6075

18. Sen B, Styner M, Xie Z et al (2009) Mechanical loading regulates NFATc1 and beta-catenin

signaling through a GSK3beta control node. J Biol Chem 284:34607–34617

19. Case N, Ma MY, Sen B et al (2008) Beta-catenin levels influence rapid mechanical responses in osteoblasts. J Biol Chem 283:29196–29205

20. Jessop HL, Rawlinson SC, Pitsillides AA et al (2002) Mechanical strain and fluid movement both activate extracellular regulated kinase (ERK) in osteoblast-like cells but via different signaling pathways. Bone 31:186–194

21. Kamel MA, Picconi JL, Lara-Castillo N et al (2010) Activation of beta-catenin signaling in MLO-Y4 osteocytic cells versus 2T3 osteoblastic cells by fluid flow shear stress and PGE2: Implications for the study of mechanosensation in bone. Bone 47:872–881

22. Rath AL, Bonewald LF, Ling J et al (2010) Correlation of cell strain in single osteocytes with intracellular calcium, but not intracellular nitric oxide, in response to fluid flow. J Biomech 43:1560–1564

23. Zaman G, Pitsillides AA, Rawlinson SC et al (1999) Mechanical strain stimulates nitric oxide production by rapid activation of endothelial nitric oxide synthase in osteocytes. J Bone Miner Res 14:1123–1131

24. Stern AR, Stern MM, Van Dyke ME et al (2012) Isolation and culture of primary osteocytes from the long bones of skeletally mature and aged mice. Biotechniques 52:361–373

25. Kitase Y, Barragan L, Qing H et al (2010) Mechanical induction of PGE2 in osteocytes blocks glucocorticoid-induced apoptosis through both the beta-catenin and PKA pathways. J Bone Miner Res 25:2657–2668

26. Genetos DC, Kephart CJ, Zhang Y et al (2007) Oscillating fluid flow activation of gap junction hemichannels induces ATP release from MLO-Y4 osteocytes. J Cell Physiol 212:207–214

27. Cherian PP, Cheng B, Gu S et al (2003) Effects of mechanical strain on the function of Gap junctions in osteocytes are mediated through the prostaglandin EP2 receptor. J Biol Chem 278:43146–43156

28. Dodds RA, Ali N, Pead MJ et al (1993) Early loading-related changes in the activity of glucose 6-phosphate dehydrogenase and alkaline phosphatase in osteocytes and periosteal osteoblasts in rat fibulae in vivo. J Bone Miner Res 8:261–267

29. Skerry TM, Bitensky L, Chayen J et al (1989) Early strain-related changes in enzyme activity in osteocytes following bone loading in vivo. J Bone Miner Res 4:783–788

30. Thompson WR, Rubin CT, Rubin J (2012) Mechanical regulation of signaling pathways in bone. Gene 503:179–193

31. Price JS, Sugiyama T, Galea GL et al (2011) Role of endocrine and paracrine factors in the adaptation of bone to mechanical loading. Curr Osteoporos Rep 9:76–82

32. Cheng M, Zaman G, Rawlinson SC et al (1999) Mechanical strain stimulates ROS cell proliferation through IGF-II and estrogen through IGF-I. J Bone Miner Res 14:1742–1750

33. Armstrong VJ, Muzylak M, Sunters A et al (2007) Wnt/beta-catenin signaling is a component of osteoblastic bone cell early responses to load-bearing and requires estrogen receptor alpha. J Biol Chem 282:20715–20727

34. Sunters A, Armstrong VJ, Zaman G et al (2010) Mechano-transduction in osteoblastic cells involves strain-regulated estrogen receptor alpha-mediated control of insulin-like growth factor (IGF) I receptor sensitivity to Ambient IGF, leading to phosphatidylinositol 3-kinase/AKT-dependent Wnt/LRP5 receptor-independent activation of beta-catenin signaling. J Biol Chem 285:8743–8758

35. Zaman G, Sunters A, Galea GL et al (2012) Loading-related regulation of the transcription factor EGR2/Krox-20 in bone cells is ERK 1/2 mediated and prostaglandin Wnt and IGF-I axis dependent. J Biol Chem 287:3946–3962

36. Zaman G, Saxon LK, Sunters A et al (2010) Loading-related regulation of gene expression in bone in the contexts of estrogen deficiency, lack of estrogen receptor alpha and disuse. Bone 46:628–642

37. Galea GL, Sunters A, Meakin LB et al (2011) Sost down-regulation by mechanical strain in human osteoblastic cells involves PGE2 signaling via EP4. FEBS Lett 585:2450–2454

38. Galea GL, Meakin LB, Sugiyama T et al (2013) Estrogen receptor alpha mediates proliferation of osteoblastic cells stimulated by estrogen and mechanical strain, but their acute down regulation of the Wnt antagonist Sost is mediated by Estrogen Receptor beta. J Biol Chem 288:9035–9048

39. Yu L, der Valk MV, Cao J et al (2011) Sclerostin expression is induced by BMPs in human Saos-2 osteosarcoma cells but not via direct effects on the sclerostin gene promoter or ECR5 element. Bone 49:1131–1140

40. Rawlinson SC, McKay IJ, Ghuman M et al (2009) Adult rat bones maintain distinct regionalized expression of markers associated with their development. PLoS One 4:e8358

41. Rawlinson SC, Mosley JR, Suswillo RF et al (1995) Calvarial and limb bone cells in organ and monolayer culture do not show the same early responses to dynamic mechanical strain. J Bone Miner Res 10:1225–1232

42. Zaman G, Suswillo RF, Cheng MZ et al (1997) Early responses to dynamic strain change and prostaglandins in bone-derived cells in culture. J Bone Miner Res 12:769–777

43. Windahl S, Saxon L, Borjesson A et al (2013) Estrogen receptor-alpha is required for the osteogenic response to mechanical loading in a ligand-independent manner involving its activation function 1 but not 2. J Bone Miner Res 28:291–301

44. Damien E, Price JS, Lanyon LE (2000) Mechanical strain stimulates osteoblast proliferation through the estrogen receptor in males as well as females. J Bone Miner Res 15: 2169–2177

45. Rubin CT, Lanyon LE (1984) Dynamic strain similarity in vertebrates; an alternative to allometric limb bone scaling. J Theor Biol 107: 321–327

Chapter 11

EPIC-μCT Imaging of Articular Cartilage

Angela S.P. Lin, Giuliana E. Salazar-Noratto, and Robert E. Guldberg

Abstract

Characterization of articular cartilage morphology and composition using microcomputed tomography (microCT) techniques requires the use of contrast agents to enhance X-ray attenuation of the tissue. This chapter describes the use of an anionic iodinated contrast agent at equilibrium with articular cartilage. In this technique, negatively charged contrast agent molecules distribute themselves inversely with respect to the negatively charged proteoglycans (PGs) within the cartilage tissue (Palmer et al. Proc Natl Acad Sci U S A 103:19255–19260, 2006). This relationship allows for assessment of cartilage degradation, as areas of high X-ray attenuation have been shown to correspond to areas of depleted PGs (Palmer et al. Proc Natl Acad Sci U S A 103:19255–19260, 2006; Xie et al. Osteoarthritis Cartilage 18:65–72, 2010).

Key words Articular cartilage, Contrast-enhanced imaging, Microcomputed tomography (micro-CT), Ionic contrast agents

1 Introduction

The current gold standard for assessing articular cartilage damage is histopathological scoring [3, 4]. However, the requisite processing and sectioning are time consuming and destructive, and only allow for semiquantitative 2D analyses that may not be representative of the 3D changes occurring within diseased joints [1]. Recent use of ionic contrast agents for enhancing X-ray attenuation of soft tissues has allowed for high-resolution 3D quantification of articular cartilage morphology and composition in small animal models of degeneration and therapeutic delivery [1, 2, 5–16]. These types of contrast-enhanced imaging techniques may facilitate development of therapeutics for degenerative joint conditions such as osteoarthritis (OA) as they can provide more rapid and more powerful 3D assessments compared to traditional histopathology.

This chapter provides a protocol for utilizing the anionic iodinated contrast agent ioxaglate (Hexabrix™, Covidien) at equilibrium with articular cartilage tissue for microCT evaluation of changes in cartilage morphology and composition. After a cartilage specimen

Jennifer J. Westendorf and Andre J. van Wijnen (eds.), *Osteoporosis and Osteoarthritis*, Methods in Molecular Biology, vol. 1226, DOI 10.1007/978-1-4939-1619-1_11, © Springer Science+Business Media New York 2015

has reached equilibrium in contrast agent solution, it is scanned, 2D slice tomograms are segmented to separate cartilage from surrounding bone and air, 3D images are generated, and quantitative parameters such as cartilage volume, average cartilage thickness, average cartilage X-ray attenuation (related to PG content), and osteophyte volume can be computed.

2   Materials

2.1   Solutions

1. Phosphate-buffered saline (PBS), without calcium and magnesium.
2. 10 % neutral buffered formalin (NBF), if tissues will be fixed before scanning.
3. PBS/protease inhibitor (PI) solution for scanning fresh tissues: Reconstitute 1× PI cocktail I (CalBiochem) crystals by adding 1 mL of PBS (without calcium and magnesium) or deionized (DI) water to PI crystals in their original vial, vortex the vial, and dilute the PI solution in PBS to make a 1 % concentration of PI in PBS (e.g., 1 mL of PI solution to 99 mL of PBS).
4. Contrast solution: Hexabrix™ in PBS (for fixed tissues) or PBS/PI solution (for fresh tissues): Create the appropriate concentration by extracting Hexabrix™ (Covidien, distributed by ASD HealthCare) with syringe and needle (18 gauge) and placing it in a conical tube that will accommodate the total volume of contrast solution needed (*see* **Note 1**). Add the appropriate volume of PBS (±PI) to Hexabrix™ in the conical tube. Vortex solution briefly until mixed. Label tube and wrap with aluminum foil (Hexabrix™ is light sensitive). Refrigerate until ready to use.

2.2   Tools and Apparatus

1. Small forceps.
2. Microdissection straight tweezers.
3. Conical tubes (15 and 50 ml).
4. Syringes and 18 gauge needles.
5. Syringe plunger (from 5 or 10 ml)—only clear plastic portion (no rubber stopper).
6. Scanco μCT40.
7. Scanco sample tube of appropriate diameter, 40 mm length.
8. Parafilm.
9. Convoluted polyurethane foam sheet (often "eggcrate" shape and charcoal color), or other material that can hold shape and prevent specimen movement in sample tube.

3   Methods

Ensure that articular cartilage surfaces are cleanly exposed and free of surrounding soft and connective tissues (including portions of ligaments). Also ensure that care is taken to prevent damage to the articular cartilage surfaces during the dissection process. The following procedures are optimized for scanning rat knee joint articular cartilage (*see* **Note 2**).

3.1   Equilibrating Specimens in Contrast Solution

1. Submerge specimen in enough contrast solution to immerse the cartilage region of interest. For rat femora, tibiae, or patellae, put 2 mL of the contrast solution in a 15 mL conical and place the specimen of interest inside. For femora, place distal end downward such that the distal articular cartilage surface is immersed in the solution. For tibiae, place proximal end downward. For patellae, immerse completely.

2. Close the conical tube and place in a water bath at 37 °C for designated equilibration time. For fresh and fixed rat tissue, this equilibration time is 30 min (*see* **Note 3**).

3. After equilibration in contrast solution, remove the specimen from the water bath and conical and pat surfaces dry with a paper towel.

3.2   Loading Specimen Securely in Scanco μCT40 Sample Tube

1. Add 0.5 ml water or PBS (without calcium and magnesium) in the bottom of a 16 mm outer diameter Scanco sample tube as a preventative measure for sample drying.

2. Wrap the specimen of interest with a small piece of polyurethane foam or other securing material in order to prevent motion of the specimen inside the sample tube.

Femur: Insert femur fully into tube, distal end up, with condyles straddling the imaginary plane created by the sample tube orientation seam (Fig. 1). This ensures that *y*-axis of scan slices will be squarely oriented in the anterior-posterior direction (axes, Fig. 1).

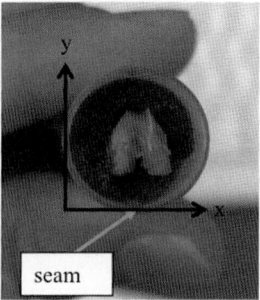

Fig. 1 Femur—Sample tube setup, *green arrow* points to orientation seam used to align the posterior aspects of the femoral condyles, *x*- and *y*-axes of resulting scan are indicated

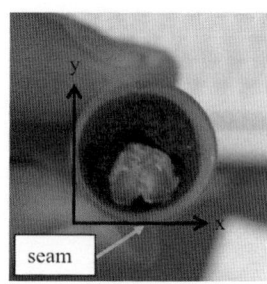

Fig. 2 Tibia—Sample tube setup, *green arrow* points to orientation seam used to align the posterior aspects of the tibial plateau, *x*- and *y*-axes of resulting scan are indicated

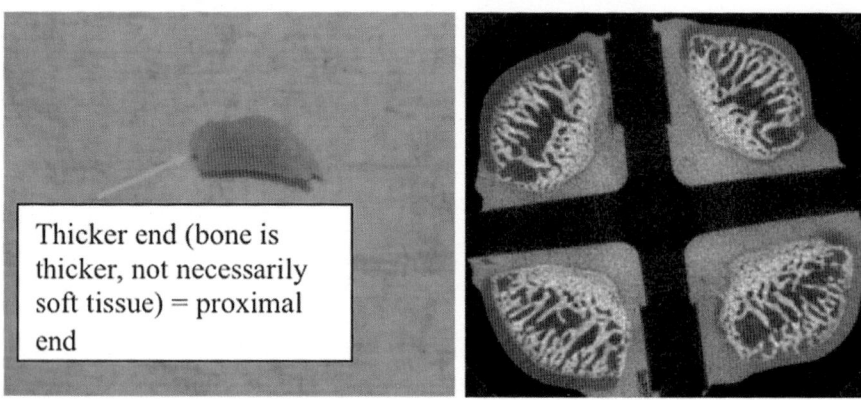

Thicker end (bone is thicker, not necessarily soft tissue) = proximal end

Fig. 3 Patella—Photograph indicating thicker/proximal end. Four patellae are positioned with proximal end upwards in sample tube, each separated by a compartment of a syringe plunger (dark cross-shaped area on sample μCT slice tomogram on the *right*)

Tibia: Insert tibia fully into tube, proximal end up, with posterior lobes straddling the imaginary plane created by the sample tube orientation seam (Fig. 2). This ensures that *y*-axis of scan slices will be squarely oriented in the anterior-posterior direction.

Patella: Vertically place four patellae within the quadrant-separating plastic portion of a syringe plunger and into the sample tube, proximal end upwards. The proximal end is thicker when looking at the patella from the side (Fig. 3).

3. Push specimen carefully below the top surface of the sample tube.

4. Cover tube opening with parafilm to seal.

3.3 Setting Scan Parameters and Running Scout View

1. Place sample tube on μCT40 stage with orientation seam facing outward.

2. Log in to the scanner's accompanying workstation, if necessary.

3. Open Tomography program via the μCT Toolbar (lower left part of the screen) (Fig. 4).

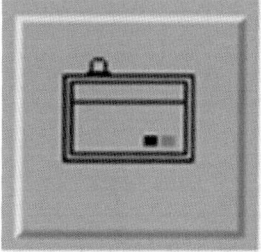

Fig. 4 Tomography Program icon in μCT Toolbar of Scanco software

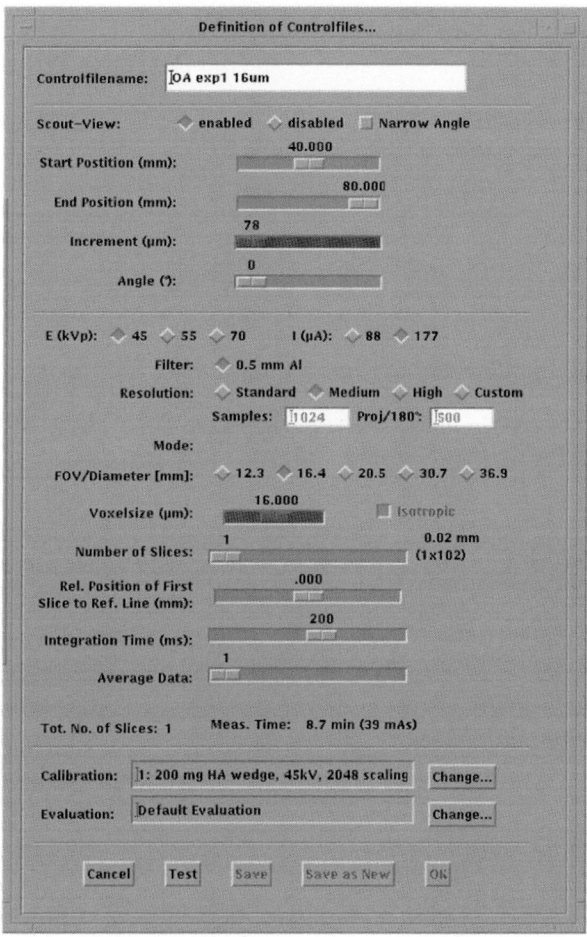

Fig. 5 Example of a scan Controlfile

4. Enter sample # when prompted (or create a new sample # if starting new set of scans).

5. Create new Controlfile with the following parameters (Fig. 5):

   • Enable Scout View with Start = 40 and End = 80 mm (*see* **Note 4**).

   • Energy $E = 45$ kVp, intensity $I = 177$ μA.

- Medium resolution ($1,024 \times 1,024$ pixel matrix).
- FOV/tube diameter 16 mm yielding 16 um voxel dimension (*see* **Note 5**).
- 200-ms integration time.
- Number of slices can be specified here or in the following steps (*see* **Note 6**).

6. In Controlfile window, click Test, then Save, and then OK.

7. Make a note of Controlfile # for future reference.

8. With appropriate sample # entered and Controlfile selected, click Scout View.

9. In Scout View window, ensure that Start Position = 40 mm, which will be near the top of the sample tube. End Position can be adjusted to any position that ensures that the cartilage region will be included (*see* **Note 7**).

10. Scout View is generated one side at a time. When complete, you will see a preview projection image of the tube contents (*see* **Note 8**).

3.4 Isolating Scan Region in Scout View Image

1. In Scout View window, click Reference Lines.

2. Bring cursor to Scout View image (green line will appear to mark the upper bound of the scan).

3. To adjust scan distance, hold Shift and drag mouse cursor without clicking any buttons. The dotted green line marks the lower bound of the scan. When the span between solid and dotted green lines marks the region of interest for the scan, release Shift.

4. Adjust the reference lines such that they include everything of interest on the specimen, and click the left mouse button to select.

5. At the bottom of the Scout View image, the number of slices, time, and length in mm will be shown—record for reference.

6. Click Scan.

7. Click Start Measurement.

8. During the scan, Tomography program will indicate the remaining time as well as show raw data sinusoids in thumbnails and preview slices in the main window (after each stack is complete).

3.5 Storing Specimen Post-imaging

1. After scanning, remove specimen from scanner.

2. Diffuse contrast solution out of tissue by placing it into the same or greater quantity of PBS or PBS/PI for the same or greater amount of time as original soak time (*see* **Note 9**).

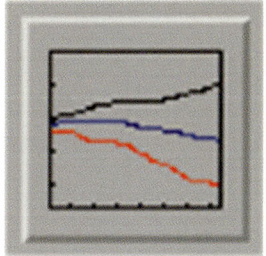

Fig. 6 Evaluation Program icon in µCT Toolbar of Scanco software

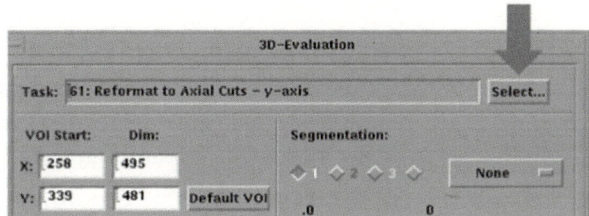

Fig. 7 3D Evaluation script selection box (click "Select…" button at *red arrow* to choose)

3.6   Evaluating the Scan Using Scanco Evaluation Software

1. Open the 3D Evaluation program from the µCT Toolbar (lower left side of the screen) (Fig. 6).

2. Select the sample and measurement number of the original scan.

3. Click Tasks → Evaluation 3D.

4. For medial-lateral direction (sagittal section) evaluations: Click "Select…" (red arrow) and in the pop-up window choose the evaluation script called Reformat Axial Slices—*y*-axis (Fig. 7) (*see* **Note 10**).

5. Resize white VOI box and relocate it (using middle and left mouse buttons on the vertices or line midpoints) such that it includes all parts of the sample.

6. Click "Start Evaluation" in the 3D Evaluation window.

7. When the evaluation completes, a new sagittally sectioned measurement number (within the same sample number) will be created.

8. Open the new reformatted file in the Evaluation program.

9. Contour the articular cartilage region in a counterclockwise direction (Fig. 8, green outline=contour) (*see* **Notes 11** and **12**).

10. Choose intensity-based segmentation parameters. Determine appropriate lower and upper threshold bounds to include cartilage tissue but exclude bone, air, and noise (*see* **Note 13**).

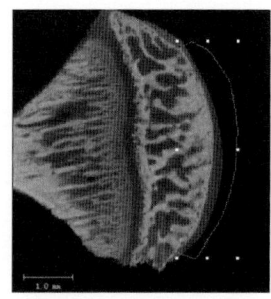

Fig. 8 Example of articular cartilage contouring (*green outline*) on a sagittal 2D slice of a rat tibial plateau

11. Evaluation scripts can be adapted to generate data including average X-ray attenuation, cartilage thickness, cartilage volume, as well as histogram text files for each.

12. Evaluations can be run on various volumes of interest by limiting slice numbers or creating different contours.

13. Original axial slices can also be resectioned to coronal slices (anterior-posterior direction) for further evaluation (using evaluation script named Reformat Axial Slices—x-axis).

4   Notes

1. For rats, 30:70 Hexabrix™:PBS solution has been typically used, and for each specimen 2 mL of contrast solution is needed. Therefore, for example, if scanning eight samples, a total volume of 16 mL contrast solution would be required (4.8 mL Hexabrix™ and 11.2 mL of PBS if you use the 30:70 ratio).

2. Sample tube size and other parameters will need to be adjusted for samples of different dimensions, composition, or diffusion and permeability characteristics.

3. Equilibration time must be determined through preliminary testing and may vary due to species, sample dimensions, diffusivity, time in fixative, and other factors.

4. If sample is large, it may be necessary to use a tube with larger diameter and height. Start position should be designated as 0 mm if using the taller tubes of height 80 mm.

5. FOV/tube diameter affects voxel size, but larger samples obviously require larger diameter tubes. Scanco μCT40 can accommodate samples up to ~34 mm diameter.

6. Other fields that may need to be adjusted: Controlfile name (top) may be changed to fit your needs. The calibration record (near the bottom) can be set to Default if you wish to display density values in linear attenuation coefficient units (1/cm).

7. Smaller difference between End Position and Start Position means shorter Scout View time.

8. If Scout View does not completely include the cartilage region, adjust the Start and/or End Positions, and re-run.

9. If fresh tissues are being tested, place specimen in fresh PBS/PI to await further processing. If fixed tissues are used, place specimen in PBS (without calcium and magnesium) to await further processing.

10. The evaluation script number (61 in the Fig. 6 example) may not match your software's numbering.

11. Boundaries between cartilage and air or subchondral bone do not need to be precise as further segmentation will be achieved through density thresholding.

12. Contouring in a clockwise direction will exclude the area within the outline. Thus, make sure to contour in a counterclockwise direction (inclusionary contours vs. exclusionary).

13. This should be conducted for several randomly selected specimens from each group before global parameters are chosen such that segmentation is consistent throughout your study.

References

1. Palmer AW, Guldberg RE, Levenston ME (2006) Analysis of cartilage matrix fixed charge density and three-dimensional morphology via contrast-enhanced microcomputed tomography. Proc Natl Acad Sci U S A 103:19255–19260

2. Xie L, Lin AS, Guldberg RE et al (2010) Nondestructive assessment of sGAG content and distribution in normal and degraded rat articular cartilage via EPIC-microCT. Osteoarthritis Cartilage 18:65–72

3. Gerwin N, Bendele AM, Glasson S et al (2010) The OARSI histopathology initiative—recommendations for histological assessments of osteoarthritis in the rat. Osteoarthritis Cartilage 18(Suppl 3):S24–S34

4. Glasson SS, Chambers MG, Van Den Berg WB et al (2010) The OARSI histopathology initiative—recommendations for histological assessments of osteoarthritis in the mouse. Osteoarthritis Cartilage 18(Suppl 3):S17–S23

5. Xie L, Lin AS, Levenston ME et al (2009) Quantitative assessment of articular cartilage morphology via EPIC-microCT. Osteoarthritis Cartilage 17:313–320

6. Xie L, Lin AS, Kundu K et al (2012) Quantitative imaging of cartilage and bone morphology, reactive oxygen species, and vascularization in a rodent model of osteoarthritis. Arthritis Rheum 64:1899–1908

7. Bansal PN, Joshi NS, Entezari V et al (2010) Contrast enhanced computed tomography can predict the glycosaminoglycan content and biomechanical properties of articular cartilage. Osteoarthritis Cartilage 18:184–191

8. Bansal PN, Joshi NS, Entezari V et al (2011) Cationic contrast agents improve quantification of glycosaminoglycan (GAG) content by contrast enhanced CT imaging of cartilage. J Orthop Res 29:704–709

9. Bansal PN, Stewart RC, Entezari V et al (2011) Contrast agent electrostatic attraction rather than repulsion to glycosaminoglycans affords a greater contrast uptake ratio and improved quantitative CT imaging in cartilage. Osteoarthritis Cartilage 19:970–976

10. Hayward LN, de Bakker CM, Gerstenfeld LC et al (2013) Assessment of contrast-enhanced computed tomography for imaging of cartilage during fracture healing. J Orthop Res 31:567–573

11. Kotwal N, Li J, Sandy J et al (2012) Initial application of EPIC-muCT to assess mouse articular cartilage morphology and composition: effects of aging and treadmill running. Osteoarthritis Cartilage 20:887–895

12. Lakin BA, Grasso DJ, Shah SS et al (2013) Cationic agent contrast-enhanced computed tomography imaging of cartilage correlates

with the compressive modulus and coefficient of friction. Osteoarthritis Cartilage 21:60–68

13. Lakin BA, Grasso DJ, Stewart RC et al (2013) Contrast enhanced CT attenuation correlates with the GAG content of bovine meniscus. J Orthop Res 31:1765–1771. doi:10.1002/jor.22421

14. Siebelt M, Waarsing JH, Kops N et al (2011) Quantifying osteoarthritic cartilage changes accurately using in vivo microCT arthrography in three etiologically distinct rat models. J Orthop Res 29:1788–1794

15. Thote T, Lin AS, Raji Y et al (2013) Localized 3D analysis of cartilage composition and morphology in small animal models of joint degeneration. Osteoarthritis Cartilage 21:1132–1141

16. Lusic H, Grinstaff MW (2013) X-ray-computed tomography contrast agents. Chem Rev 113:1641–1666

Part IV

In Vivo Models of Disease and Repair

Chapter 12

Mouse Models of Osteoarthritis: Surgical Model of Posttraumatic Osteoarthritis Induced by Destabilization of the Medial Meniscus

Kirsty L. Culley, Cecilia L. Dragomir, Jun Chang, Elisabeth B. Wondimu, Jonathan Coico, Darren A. Plumb, Miguel Otero, and Mary B. Goldring

Abstract

The surgical model of destabilization of the medial meniscus (DMM) has become a gold standard for studying the onset and progression of posttraumatic osteoarthritis (OA). The DMM model mimics clinical meniscal injury, a known predisposing factor for the development of human OA, and permits the study of structural and biological changes over the course of the disease. In addition, when applied to genetically modified or engineered mouse models, this surgical procedure permits dissection of the relative contribution of a given gene to OA initiation and/or progression. This chapter describes the requirements for the surgical induction of OA in mouse models, and provides guidelines and tools for the subsequent histological, immunohistochemical, and molecular analyses. Methods for the assessment of the contributions of selected genes in genetically modified strains are also provided.

Key words Surgical model, Histology, Immunohistochemistry, RNA extraction

1 Introduction

Osteoarthritis (OA) is a "whole joint" disorder involving all joint tissues, with progressive cartilage erosion as the major pathological indicator leading to joint replacement surgery. Posttraumatic osteoarthritis (PTOA) represents a subset of OA in which the end stage of the disease may be very similar to idiopathic OA, but the initial causes, stages of development and progression, patient populations, and potential approaches to therapy are distinct. Biomechanical instability of the joint is one of the known risk factors in the pathogenesis of OA, and is the prevalent factor involved in the development of PTOA, in particular. Over the years we have gained understanding of the molecular mechanisms driving the destruction of cartilage and other joint tissues in OA, based on analyses of gene and protein expression in clinical material and in cell

Jennifer J. Westendorf and Andre J. van Wijnen (eds.), *Osteoporosis and Osteoarthritis*, Methods in Molecular Biology, vol. 1226, DOI 10.1007/978-1-4939-1619-1_12, © Springer Science+Business Media New York 2015

culture models derived from human tissues. However, we currently have no disease-modifying OA drug (DMOAD) partly because observations in human joint tissues in situ can be made only in retrieved surgical or postmortem specimens. Therefore, following human patients longitudinally during the development of OA disease is not possible. Furthermore, biomarkers in synovial fluid, serum, and urine, as well as MRI, have yet to be fully characterized for early diagnosis or therapeutic outcome in cohorts, let alone in individual patients.

No OA animal model is entirely predictive of human responses, and it still remains unclear how well any of the available models resemble idiopathic OA in the aging human population. Spontaneous OA models such as the Str/ort mouse [1] are available and widely used. However, the long time course of disease development over several months makes the spontaneous models less attractive for examining the effects of therapies. A noninvasive tibial loading model has recently been developed and represents an attractive alternative for replicating OA in the mouse because both cartilage and bone changes occur in a defined manner both spatially and temporally [2, 3]. Mouse models with the same mutations as in human chondrodysplasias develop OA with age due to abnormal composition and structure of joint tissues, such as articular cartilage, and associated biomechanical instability. The molecular phenotypes resemble those reported in the profiling studies of human cartilage [4, 5], in which both catabolic and anabolic gene signatures have been identified.

Surgical models of PTOA, in which the ACL or other knee ligaments are transected in different animal species, reflect many aspects of PTOA in humans and have several advantages over spontaneous models, including faster disease onset, decreased genetic drift, and better reproducibility. Surgical instability models in dog, guinea pig, rabbit, rat, sheep, and goat are all used widely to replicate aspects of human OA disease. Due to the high cost of maintaining larger species and the availability of genetically modified strains, surgical PTOA models in mice are preferred for preliminary screening and for determining the in vivo influence of knockout or transgenic overexpression of a given gene on the initiation and progression of disease throughout a time course of several weeks [6, 7]. Indeed, genetically modified mice and different mouse strains are employed to uncover mechanisms associated with risk factors such as biomechanical instability, injury, inflammation, obesity, and genetic mutations and permit gene profiling over the time course of OA initiation and progression [8–12]. Although aging does not inevitably lead to OA, age-related responses in joint tissues of different mouse strains are accelerated in PTOA models [11]. Common to all mouse models of OA are certain molecular pathways, particularly those controlling expression and activation of proteolytic enzymes, which determine initiation and progression of cartilage damage. Together, the findings to date suggest that the OA signature may be disease-specific and unrelated to aging. These findings therefore lend credence to the possibility of identifying gene signatures in at-risk populations, including those susceptible to PTOA, prior to the onset of overt OA.

The surgical model of destabilization of the medial meniscus (DMM) has become a gold standard in the field. DMM surgery was used to demonstrate the importance of the key aggrecan- and collagen-degrading enzymes in cartilage destruction in mice deficient in *Adamts5* [13, 14] and *Mmp13* [15]. Reduced severity of OA, and in some cases increased regeneration, were demonstrated in PTOA mouse or rat models treated with a syndecan-4 antibody [16], a Hedgehog signaling inhibitor [17], recombinant human PTH(1–34) (teriparatide) [18], an aggrecanase inhibitor [19], and kartogenin, a small molecule targeting the chondrogenic program [20]. Glasson [6] highlighted the importance of murine genetic background in PTOA models while screening several mouse strains in the DMM model. The 129/SvEv mice are most susceptible to surgical OA induction, whereas the least susceptible strain tested is DBA/1, which is highly susceptible to autoimmune or inflammatory arthritis. The C57BL/6 strain, used most frequently for generation of knockout and transgenic mice, either alone or on a mixed background with 129/SvDv strains, has intermediate susceptibility, indicating its utility in determining whether the chosen genetic modification is expected to enhance or attenuate cartilage loss following challenge. More recent studies using a population genetics approach to generate recombinant inbred mouse strains have also highlighted the concept that strain-related differences in mice may reflect OA susceptibility differences in humans. These studies comparing strains derived from the MRL/MpJ superhealer mouse with different healing capacities [21, 22] showed inverse correlation between cartilage healing and OA development in a PTOA model.

In this chapter, we provide detailed methodology and guidelines to conduct the DMM surgical model, with special emphasis on the histological, immunohistochemical, and molecular analyses for evaluation of the impact on the development and progression of OA.

2 Materials

2.1 Conditional Deletion or Induction of Transgene Expression in Genetically Modified Mice

2.1.1 Tamoxifen Treatment for Deletion of Floxed Alleles

1. Tamoxifen powder.

2. Sunflower seed oil from *Helianthus annus*.

3. Ethanol.

4. 1/2 cc Tuberculin syringe with 27-gauge ½-in needle.

5. 2 cc Lactated Ringer Injection USP solution.

6. 10 or 20 mL Luer-Lok Tip syringe and 25-gauge 5/8-in needle.

7. DietGel Recovery, Purified Dietary Supplement for Laboratory Rodents (Fisher and Son, NJ).

2.1.2 Doxycycline
Treatment for Control
of Tetracycline-Regulated
Promoters

1. Doxycycline Hyclate powder.
2. Autoclaved water.

2.2 Anesthesia
Induction
and Maintenance

1. 2 cc Lactated Ringer Injection USP solution.
2. 10 mL Luer-Lok Tip syringe and 25-gauge 5/8-in needle.
3. Ketamine at 30 mg/kg of body weight (Ketaset, 100 mg/mL).
4. Xylazine at 5 mg/kg of body weight (Rompun, 20 mg/mL).
5. Acetylpromazine at 1 mg/kg body weight (Acepromazine, 10 mg/mL).
6. 1/2 cc Tuberculin syringe with 27-gauge 1/2-in needle.
7. Buprenorphine at 0.5 mg/kg of body weight (Buprenex, 0.3 mg/mL).
8. 1/2 cc Tuberculin syringe with 27-gauge 1/2-in needle.

2.3 Preparation
of Surgical Site

1. Hazard Technology Golden A5 Electric Hair Clippers attached to a containment vacuum with HEPA filter (Oster Professional, McMinnville, TN).
2. 4 % Chlorhexidine Gluconate Surgical Brush/Sponge (BD Company, NJ).
3. 70 % Isopropyl Alcohol.
4. Gauze Sponges.

2.4 Surgical
Reagents
and Equipment

All surgical tools must be sterilized prior to surgery.

1. Zeiss Surgical Microscope, Super Lux 40.
2. Surgical Blades; size 11 and size 15.
3. Q-tips.
4. Mini dissecting Scissors (World Precision Instruments, Sarasota, FL).
5. Student Vannas Scissors (World Precision Instruments, Sarasota, FL).
6. Dumont Tweezers #5B, 45° angled (World Precision Instruments, Sarasota, FL).
7. Dumont Tweezers #5, straight (World Precision Instruments, Sarasota, FL).
8. Tyrell Hook (World Precision Instruments, Sarasota, FL).
9. Micro Castroviejo Needle Holder (World Precision Instruments, Sarasota, FL).
10. 2× Feather Scalpel Handles #3 (Electron Microscopy Sciences, Hatfield, PA).

11. Coated Vicryl Suture (8-0 (0.4 metric) 12″ (30 cm) TG140-8 6.5 mm 3/8c) (Ethicon Inc., Somerville, NJ).

12. VETClose Surgical Adhesive containing formulated cyanoacrylate (Henry Schein Animal Health, Dublin, Ohio).

13. 0.9 % Sodium Chloride irrigation USP Solution.

14. Powdered Sterile Surgical Gloves.

15. Sterile Surgical Gown.

16. Sterile Gauze Sponges.

2.5 Mouse Housing

Housing of mice at four mice per cage in large cages, according to NIH and IACUC guidelines will maintain a level of activity that will induce OA postoperatively.

1. Thoren Ventilated Rack (Thoren Caging Sytems Inc., Hazelton, PA).

2. Thoren weaning cages (model #2, polycarbonate, dimensions: L12.125 × W12.125 × H5.625, Thoren Caging Systems Inc., Hazelton, PA).

3. Polished stainless steel wire for mice cages (Thoren Caging Sytems Inc., Hazelton, PA).

4. Nestpacks, Betachip, 100gr Bedding (Fisher and Son, NJ).

5. LabDiet 5053 irradiated, PicoLab Rodent Diet 20 (Fisher and Son, NJ).

6. DietGel Recovery, Purified Dietary Supplement for Laboratory Rodents (Fisher and Son, NJ).

7. Mouse Tunnels (BioServ Frenchtown, NJ).

2.6 Sample Fixation, Decalcification, and Processing

2.6.1 Tissue Fixation

1. 10× Phosphate-Buffered Solution (PBS).

2. 4 % paraformaldehyde (PFA): Heat 400 mL of 1× dH_2O to 60 °C and add 20 g of PFA while stirring. Add 500 µL of 2 N NaOH and continue to stir until the PFA goes into solution. Add 50 mL of 10× PBS, and add dH_2O water to final volume of 500 mL; bring to pH 7.4 with hydrochloric acid. Filter the solution through a 0.45 µM filter. Aliquot and freeze at −20 °C for long-term storage.

3. 2 N sodium hydroxide: Dissolve 4 g of NaOH pellets in 40 mL dH_2O; make to a final volume of 50 mL.

4. Hydrochloric Acid.

5. 0.45 µM Filter.

6. 15 mL Falcon tubes or Tissue- Tek Biopsy Uni-Casettes (Sakura, Torrance, CA).

7. Rocker.

2.6.2 Tissue Decalcification

1. *20 % sodium citrate dihydrate*: dissolve 100 g of sodium citrate dihydrate in 350 mL of dH$_2$O; add dH$_2$O to a final volume of 500 mL.

2. *45 % formic acid*: To prepare 500 mL dilute 225 mL of >95 % formic acid in 275 mL of dH$_2$O.

3. *2 N sodium hydroxide*: Dissolve 4 g of NaOH pellets in 40 mL dH$_2$O; make to a final volume of 50 mL.

4. *10 % EDTA*: Add 100 g of EDTA to 850 mL dH$_2$O while stirring. Adjust the final volume to 1 L with dH$_2$O and pH to 7.4 using sodium hydroxide pellets.

5. *Ammonium oxalate monohydrate (AO):* Weigh 10 g of AO and add to 150–200 mL of dH$_2$O whilst stirring. Heat gently to dissolve all the ammonium sulfate and continue to add AO until the solution becomes saturated. Precipitates of ammonium sulfate crystals should form and will indicate that the solution is fully saturated. Allow the solution to cool to room temperature before use.

2.6.3 Tissue Processing

1. Tissue-Tek Biopsy Uni-Cassette (Sakura, Torrance, CA).

2. Specimen Foam Pads (Electron Microscopy Sciences, Hatfield, PA).

3. Ethanol.

4. Xylene.

5. Paraffin.

6. Spin Tissue Processor (Model STP120) (ThermoFisher Scientific Microm, Rockford, IL).

7. Tissue Embedding Center (Model EC350-1) (ThermoFisher Scientific Microm, Rockford, IL).

8. Base Molds (Electron Microscopy Sciences, Hatfieldd, PA).

2.6.4 Sectioning

1. HM 355S Automatic Microtome.

2. MX35 Ultra Blades (Richard-Allan Scientific, Kalamazoo, MI).

3. Diamond White Glass microscope slides.

4. 37 °C Oven.

5. Slide storage file.

2.7 Histological Staining

1. Xylene.

2. Ethanols: 70, 80, 90, and 100 %.

3. 10× Phosphate-Buffered Solution (PBS).

4. *Shandon instant hematoxylin solution*: Prepare the day before staining following manufacturer's instructions. Briefly, mix one bottle of part A and one bottle of part B in 1 L of dH$_2$O and

stir overnight at room temperature. Filter the hematoxylin solution through chromatography paper before every use. After preparation, the hematoxylin solution can be stored at room temperature and reused for up to 1 month.

5. *Scott's buffer solution*: Add 10 g of magnesium sulfate and 2 g of sodium bicarbonate to 1 L of dH_2O and stir for 30 min before using. Prepare freshly for every staining.

6. Fast Green 0.2 % Solution.

7. *1 % acetic acid solution*: Add 10 mL of glacial acetic acid to 90 mL of dH_2O. Prepare freshly for every use.

8. Safranin O 0.5 % Solution.

9. VectaMount (Vector Laboratories Inc., Burlingame, CA).

10. SuperSlip CoverGlass 20×50×1.

11. Slide storage file.

12. Chromatography paper.

2.8 Immunohisto-chemistry (IHC) and Immunofluo-rescence (IF)

IHC and IF conditions (e.g., retrieval method, or primary and secondary antibody concentration) may vary and require optimization. The provided protocols are guidelines and have been optimized for the specified antibodies utilizing the reagents indicated.

1. Xylene.

2. Ethanol.

3. 1× Phosphate-Buffered Solution (PBS).

4. Antigen retrieval of choice (e.g., 2 mg/mL hyaluronidase).

5. 3 % H_2O_2 (required for IHC only).

6. Humid Chamber.

7. Liquid Blocker, Super Pap Pen Mini (Ted Pella Inc., Redding, CA).

8. Blocking solution.

9. Primary Antibody.

10. Secondary Antibody (e.g., Biotinylated Ab Vectastain ABC Elite Kits, Vector Laboratories Inc., Burlingame, CA; Abcam, Cambridge, MA; or Alexa Fluor Molecular Probes Cell Signaling, Billerica, MA).

11. Tween-20.

12. Avidin/Biotin Reagent (Vectastain ABC Elite Kits, Vector Laboratories Inc., Burlingame, CA) (required for IHC only).

13. DAB Chromogen (DAKO, CA) or Vector NovaRED (Vector Laboratories Inc., Burlingame, CA) (required for immunohistochemistry only).

14. 0.2 % Fast Green solution.

15. VectaMount (Vector Laboratories Inc., Burlingame, CA) required for immunohistochemistry only.

16. ProLong Gold antifade reagent with DAPI (Molecular Probes by Life Technologies Corp., Eugene, OR) (required for immunofluorescence only).

17. SuperSlip CoverGlass 20×50×1.

18. Slide storage file.

2.9 RNA Extraction and Gene Expression Analysis of Mouse Articular Cartilage

2.9.1 Isolation of Articular Cartilage

1. Sterile Phosphate-buffered saline (PBS) (Cell culture standard); ice-cold for dissecting mouse knees.

2. Dissecting scissors.

3. Straight forceps (Hampton Research, Aliso Viejo, CA).

4. Curved tipped forceps (Hampton Research, Aliso Viejo, CA).

5. Two star quality micro scissors 3″ blade.

6. Stereo zoom microscope.

7. Microscope stand with focus mount.

8. Nova 2000 fiber optic illuminator and optic guides (Nikon, Melville, NY).

9. 2× Feather Scalpel handle # 3.

10. Surgical Blades; size 11 and size 15.

11. RNAlater (Ambion Life technologies, Grand Island, NY).

12. DNase/RNase-free Eppendorf tubes.

13. Filter pipette tips (Nuclease-free).

2.9.2 Total RNA Isolation from Cartilage Using a Modified mirVana™ Protocol

1. TRIzol® Reagent (Invitrogen, Grand Island, NY).

2. QIAshredder (Qiagen Inc., Valencia, CA).

3. Chloroform:Isoamyl alcohol (IAA) 24:1.

4. Phenol:chloroform:IAA, 125:24:1.

5. Molecular-grade ethanol, nuclease-free.

6. *Mir*Vana miRNA Isolation Kit, without phenol (Ambion Life Technologies, Grand Island, NY).

7. DNA-free Kit (Ambion Life Technologies, Grand Island, NY).

8. 3 M Sodium Acetate pH 5.5, nuclease-free.

9. UltraPure Glycogen, nuclease-free.

10. Nuclease-free water.

11. Hand-held homogenizer (VWR Pellet Mixer) (VWR International, Radnor, PA).

12. Nuclease-free pestles (Argos Technologies, Elgin, IL).

13. NanoDrop spectrophotometer (ThermoFisher Scientific Inc., Rockford, IL).

14. Bioanalyzer (Agilent Technologies, Santa Clara, CA).

3   Methods

3.1   Conditional Deletion or Induction of Transgene Expression in Genetically Modified Mice

3.1.1   Tamoxifen Treatment of Mice for Conditional Gene Ablation

Although global knockout models have been used in combination with the DMM surgery to uncover the contributions of proteins such as aggrecanases [13] and collagenase [15] to cartilage degradation, gene modifications frequently present developmental alterations that add confounding factors and extra complexity. Thus, inducible models, in which a gene can be knocked-out in a specific tissue at a desired time-point, have been developed. To determine if conditional ablation of a gene in cartilage affects the onset and/or progression of PTOA, mice containing the floxed alleles of the gene of interest are crossed with mice harboring cartilage-specific inducible Cre recombinase transgenes, such as the minimal *Col2a1* promoter transgenes (*Col2a1*-Cre-ER [23] or *Col2a1*-Cre-ER^{T2} [24] or the targeted *Agc1* (*aggrecan*)-*CreER^{T2}* knockin allele [25, 26]. These inducible Cre strains contain a transgene that expresses a modified form of Cre recombinase, which is controlled by a mutated version of the mouse estrogen receptor ligand-binding domain, which does not bind natural estrogen at physiological concentrations, but instead binds the estrogen-derivative tamoxifen. Therefore, administration of tamoxifen at a desired time point allows elucidation of the role of a gene at different stages of embryonic development, after birth, or in adult life. Described below is one method of tamoxifen administration for Cre-recombinase-mediated deletion of floxed genes in adult mice prior to DMM surgery.

3.1.2   Tamoxifen Administration by Intraperitoneal Injection

1. Dissolve 30 mg of tamoxifen in 100 μL ethanol and vortex for 5 min.

2. Add 900 μL of sunflower oil and incubate at 37 °C to improve solubility; it should be completely dissolved in approximately 1 h with periodic vortexing to speed up the process.

3. Aliquot the tamoxifen for storage. Store at 4 °C for 2 weeks (maximum) or at −20 °C for months.

4. Administer medications intraperitoneally into the right lower abdominal quadrant, with the animal's anterior body tilted down, via 0.5-cc tuberculin syringe with a 27-gauge 1/2-in. needle. To facilitate access to food and water, recovery gel cups and food pellets are placed on the floor of the cage with the mice.

5. At the time of tamoxifen injection, administer 2 cc of lactated Ringer's solution subcutaneously to each mouse using a 10 mL Luer-Lok Tip syringe and 25-gauge 5/8-in needle (*see* **Note 1**).

3.1.3   Doxycycline Treatment for Tetracycline-Inducible Transgene Expression

The tetracycline-controlled transcriptional activation Tet-Off system [27] is widely used to achieve expression of transgenes controlled by tissue-specific promoters. The Tet-Off system requires a responder construct (containing a tetracycline-responsive element,

TRE) that controls the expression of the transgene of interest, and an activator construct (with a Tet-controlled transcriptional activator, tTA). Binding of tTA to the TRE induces transcription of a specific gene downstream of TRE. In the Tet-Off system, when doxycycline is present it binds to tTA to prevent it from binding to the TRE. However, when doxycycline is absent, tTA binds to the TRE and activates tissue-specific transcription of the gene of interest localized downstream of TRE. To study the effects of the inducible overexpression of a given gene, use murine strains that express tTA under the control of cartilage-specific promoters, such as *Col2a1* [28] or *Comp* [29].

3.1.4 Doxycycline Administration (See **Note 2***)*

1. Prepare doxycycline at a concentration of 1 mg/mL in drinking water.

2. Administer doxycycline orally, ad libitum, to female pregnant mice.

3. Change water and doxycycline weekly.

4. Continue the treatment during the entire pregnancy period, and until weaning at 1 month after birth.

5. At 1 month after birth, remove doxycycline from the drinking water to induce transgene expression. The expression level of the transgene must be determined empirically prior to the completion of DMM surgery.

3.2 Surgical Resection of Mouse Knee Joints

DMM surgery (*see* **Note 3**) is performed, generally in 12-week-old mice, as described previously by Glasson et al. [30]. Briefly, unilateral joint instability is induced by microsurgical transection of the medial meniscotibial ligament (MMTL), which anchors the medial meniscus to the tibial plateau (*see* **Note 4**). DMM surgery is completed in the right knee, leaving the left knee as a nonoperated control or a sham-operated control, in which the meniscotibial ligament is localized but not transected (*see* **Note 5**).

1. Administer to mice subcutaneously 2 cc of lactated Ringer solution prior to anesthesia using a 10 mL Luer-Lok Tip syringe and 25-gauge 5/8-in needle.

2. Administer medications (ketamine, xylazine and acetylpromazine) by intraperitoneal injection into the right lower abdominal quadrant, with the anterior body tilted down, via a ½ cc tuberculin syringe with a 27-gauge 1/2-in. needle. This single dose provides 15–20 min of surgical anesthesia. If necessary, anesthesia may be prolonged by administration of isoflurane gas via a nose cone.

3. Use electrical hair clippers to remove hair from the surgical site. Prepare the site by scrubbing twice with a 4 % chlorhexidine surgical brush/sponge, and then wiping with 70 % isopropyl alcohol.

4. Perform arthrotomy to expose the femoral tibial joint. Make a longitudinal incision of approximately 5 mm over the distal patellar tendon to the proximal tibial plateau.

5. Incise the joint capsule immediately medial to the patellar tendon with a size 15 blade, and gently lift the tendon with 45° Dumont tweezers to allow access of the Tyrell hook by technician. Use the Tyrell hook to move the tendon to one side to allow access to the joint compartment.

6. Optional (*see* **Note 6**): Perform blunt dissection of the fat pad over the intercondylar area using 45° Dumont tweezer to expose the medial meniscotibial ligament (MMTL). Control mild hemorrhaging from the fat pad by applying pressure with Q-tips.

7. Identify the MMTL running from the cranial horn of the medial meniscus laterally onto the anterior tibial plateau. Take care to identify and avoid the lateral meniscotibial ligament (LMTL), which is posterior and has fibers running in a similar direction.

8. Section the MMTL with a size 11 blade, with the blade directed proximo-laterally to destabilize the medial meniscus. Use the 45° Dumont tweezer to check if the MMTL is fully transected and the medial meniscus destabilized.

9. Suture close the joint capsule and subcutaneous layer with Coated Vicryl Suture (8-0) and close the skin by application of VETClose Surgical Adhesive If the joint tissues become dry at any point prior to suturing, rehydrate with 0.9 % sodium chloride USP solution.

10. Immediately after anesthetic recovery administer an initial dose of buprenorphine (Buprenex 0.3 mg/mL) at 0.05 mg/kg subcutaneously. Place mice in cages that are maintained on warming blankets and continue to monitor until the mice are awake. Administer buprenorphine at 0.05 mg/kg subcutaneously every 8–12 h (or more frequently if needed) for a duration of 48 h postoperatively [31]. Analgesic support may be extended for certain procedures as deemed by the IACUC and/or veterinary input. Additional analgesia may be given at the discretion of the veterinary staff. Routinely after short procedures, mice are ambulatory and appetent. Animals that are inappetent, nonambulatory, or manifest any other sign of illness (porphyria, poor hair coat, weight loss, etc.) are examined and appropriate therapy is administered (e.g. antibiotics, fluid therapy, additional analgesic, warming pad, or euthanasia if necessary) (*see* **Note 7**).

11. Place an unopened nest pack containing bedding (*see* **Note 8**) and a mouse tunnel (to promote activity) (*see* **Note 9**) in the cage and allow mice to move in their cages ad lib. For the first 48

postoperative hours, to facilitate access to food and water, recovery gel cups and food pellets are placed on the floor of the cage. Animals are assessed by veterinary staff on the second postoperative day. Prophylactic or postoperative antibiotics are not administered routinely for short procedures performed under aseptic conditions.

12. Optional: Assess the effects of drugs or other reagents on the course of OA development and progression postsurgery by comparing the agent versus the vehicle in different groups of DMM-operated animals (the number of animals required per treatment group for histological analysis is determined by power analysis). For a single-dosing regimen, administer to separate knees the agent or vehicle (e.g., PBS) at 1 or 2 weeks postsurgery (pre-onset OA), or if one injection is not sufficient, dosing at 1–3 times per week over a subsequent 4-week period may be attempted. Additionally drugs can delivered/administered systemically via methods such as introduction into the diet or via osmotic pumps implanted subcutaneously.

3.3 Histological Assessment of OA pathology

The animals are sacrificed (according to IACUC guidelines) (*see* **Note 10**) at appropriate time points post-DMM surgery and the knee joints collected for histological assessment to determine the effects of time or genotype on experimental OA. The pathology is assessed using a modified Mankin scoring system recommended by OARSI [32] based on Safranin O-stained histological sections. Meniscus, subchondral bone, and osteophyte formation may also be examined in the same sections to evaluate the overall condition of the joints. Guidelines and examples for sample processing in order to complete histological evaluation are provided in the following sections.

3.3.1 Fixation

1. Immediately after sacrifice dissect knees for histological analysis and remove skin and excess muscle with dissection scissors. Trim the femur and tibia so that they are ~0.5-in. in length (*see* Fig. 1), then place the dissected knees in individual falcon tubes or biopsy cassettes for tissue fixation in 4 % PFA. It is advisable that the volume of PFA (or other fixative) is at least 15–20× the volume of tissue.

2. Fix samples for the desired length of time depending on your antibody/staining to be completed downstream (duration of fixation is based on previous standardized histology or immunohistochemistry (IHC)/immunofluorescence (IF). During fixation, place samples on a rocker or shaker.

3. Following fixation, wash the samples with dH_2O for 1 h at room temperature on a shaker, changing the dH_2O every 15 min.

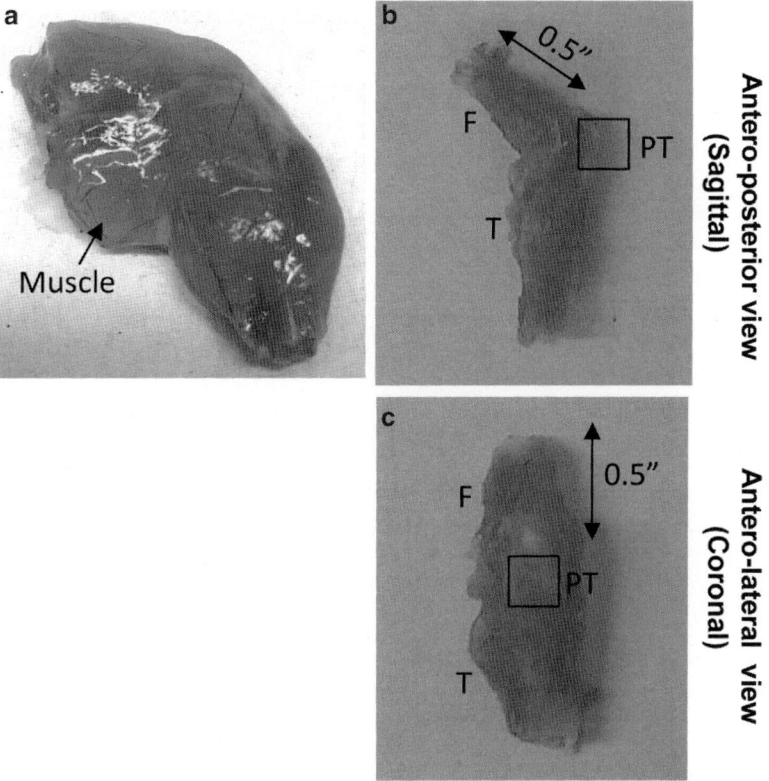

Fig. 1 Trimming mouse knee joints for embedding in paraffin. Once the leg has been dissected (**a**) it is important to remove as much muscle (M) as possible (**b** and **c**) to prevent the knee from bending during processing. The tibia (T) and femur (F) should be cut to approximately 0.5 in. with the patellar tendon (PT) located in the center of the specimen

3.3.2 Decalcification

There are several available methods for decalcification and, while the appropriate method should be selected based on the subsequent histological/immunohistochemical analyses, it should remain consistent within each experimental model studied. Depending on the method selected, the time required for decalcification and subsequent retrieval method for immunostaining will change. In this section we will detail two methods for decalcification (EDTA and formic acid:sodium citrate), both of which are suitable for reliable Safranin O/Fast green staining and scoring. Other available methods include, but are not limited to, 5–10 % nitric acid or 10 % HCl.

Sodium Citrate/Formic Acid Decalcification

1. Mix 250 mL of 45 % formic acid with 250 mL of 20 % sodium citrate dihydrate solution. Add decalcification solution to sample. The recommended volume of decalcification solution is at least 15–20× the volume of tissue.

2. Incubate samples at room temperature on a rocker for 2–3 days.

3. Assess samples to determine if they are decalcified after 2–3 days (*see* the decalcification test below using a solution of saturated ammonium oxalate).

4. Change the 45 % formic acid/ 20 % sodium citrate dihydrate fixation solution for fresh solution every 3 days. The decalcification should be complete within in approximately 5–7 days.

10 % EDTA Decalcification

1. Add 10 % EDTA, pH 7.4 to samples; the recommended volume of decalcification solution is at least 15–20× the volume of tissue.

2. Incubate samples on a rocker at room temperature for 3–14 days, changing the solution two times per week.

Decalcification Test

1. Take 1 mL of the decalcification solution from the samples that you are decalcifying and add 5 mL of saturated AO solution. Mix well, incubate for 30 min at room temperature, and check for a white precipitate by holding against a black background.

2. If a white precipitate forms, remove the decalcification solution from the samples and add fresh decalcification solution. Incubate the samples for 2–3 more days at room temperature on a shaker. Decalcification is complete only if no white precipitate is formed.

3. Once decalcification is complete, wash samples in dH_2O for a minimum of 6 h. Change the water every 30 min or place samples (in biopsy cassettes) under a gentle flow of clean running water.

4. After washing, place the samples in 70 % ethanol for temporary storage at 4 °C until ready for embedding (long-term storage at 4 °C is not recommended) (*see* **Note 11**).

3.3.3 Processing and Embedding

1. Place samples in Tissue-Tek Biopsy Uni-Cassettes, if not already done so. Use two specimen foam pads to stabilize the joint in the cassette if the mouse knee is too small.

2. Process samples using a tissue processor with the following guidelines: 70 % ETOH (7 h or overnight), followed by 80 % EtOH (1 h), 90 % EtOH (1 h), 100 % EtOH (3× each for 1 h), Xylene (2× each for 1.5 h), and paraffin (2× each for 2 h).

3. Embed samples in fresh paraffin in tissue molds using a tissue-embedding station. Allow paraffin to set, remove samples from molds, and store long-term at 4 °C (*see* Fig. 2 for orientation of knee for coronal sections and Fig. 3 for sagittal sections).

3.3.4 Sectioning

1. Cut serial coronal sections of 6 μm throughout the whole embedded mouse knee joint using a microtome (*see* **Note 12**).

2. Mount three sections per Diamond White Glass microscope slides.

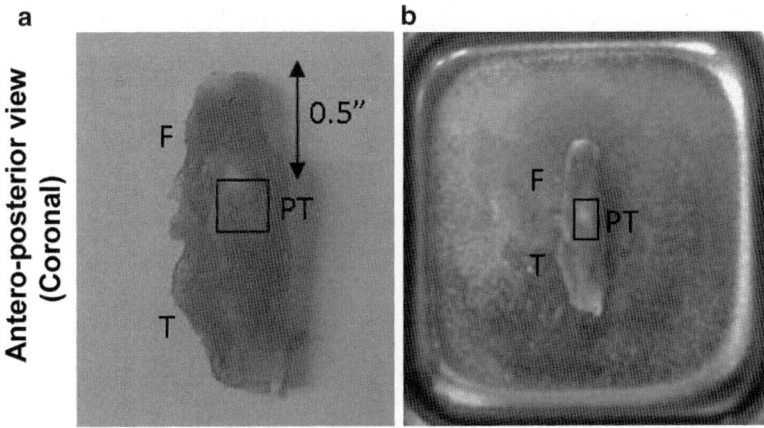

Fig. 2 Orientation of mouse knee joints for paraffin-embedded coronal sections. (**a**) Coronal view of the trimmed knee with the patellar tendon (PT) is easily visualized. (**b**) The specimen is placed in a metallic mold ready for paraffin embedding. For coronal sectioning, orient the femur (F) facing upwards and the tibia (T) downwards in relation to the mold, using forceps to ensure that the patellar tendon is facing up and centered within the mold

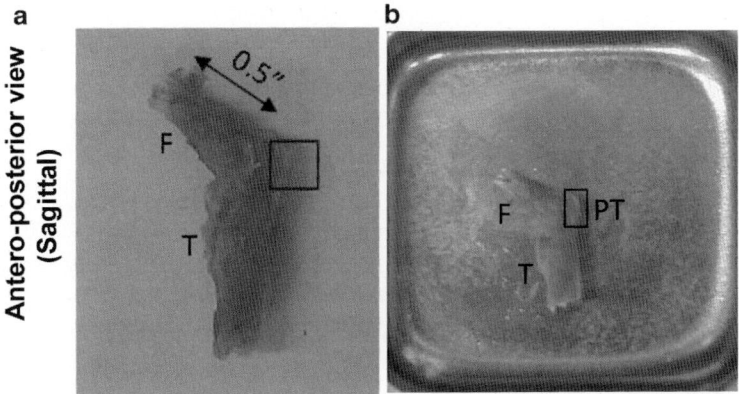

Fig. 3 Orientation of mouse knee joints for paraffin-embedded sagittal sections. (**a**) Sagittal view of the trimmed knee with the patellar tendon (PT) is easily visualized. (**b**) The specimen is placed in a metallic mold ready for paraffin embedding. For sagittal sectioning, orient the femur (F) and tibia (T) so they are facing left in relation to the mold, using forceps to ensure that the patellar tendon is facing to the right and the sample is centered in the mold

3. Allow slides to dry overnight in a 37 °C oven to remove any water that may be trapped under sections.

4. Stain every fifth slide (every 90 μm) with Safranin O for OA histological scoring, leaving intervening slides for immunohistochemistry or immunofluorescence.

Optional: Prior to completing staining protocols, paraffin-embedded sections can be placed on a slide heating block at 60 °C overnight.

*3.3.5 Histological
Staining*

1. Deparaffinize in Xylene 2× for 8 min each (in the fume hood).

2. Rehydrate in an ethanol series: 100 % EtOH (2×, 5 min each); 95 % EtOH (5 min); 85 % EtOH (4 min); and 70 % EtOH (4 min).

3. Incubate slides in filtered hematoxylin for 30 s.

4. Rinse slides in tap water three times for 5 min each until water is clear.

5. Incubate in Scott's Buffer for 2 min.

6. Rinse slides in tap water three times for 5 min each.

7. Incubate in 0.2 % Fast green for 4 min.

8. Rinse quickly in 1 % acetic acid solution (dip three times).

9. Rinse quickly in tap water.

10. Stain slides in 0.5 % Safranin O for 5 min.

11. Rinse slides in 95 % EtOH (dip three times).

12. Rinse slides in100 % EtOH (dip three times).

13. Incubate slides in 100 % EtOH for approximately 2 min. If the ethanol is still pink after 2 min, place the slides in a fresh ethanol bath for another minute.

14. Incubate slides in Xylene for 3 min followed by fresh Xylene for 10 min (in the fume hood).

15. Mount sections with Vectamount medium and SuperSlip CoverGlass.

*3.3.6 Histological
Scoring*

A well-established histological scoring system, which utilizes Safranin O-stained sections (*see* Fig. 4 for a representative section identifying joint structures), serves as the primary outcome measure to determine the rate and extent of OA in the DMM model. Due to the thin nature of mouse articular cartilage, a modified Mankin histological grading scale recommended in the OARSI Histopathology Atlas by Glasson et al. [32] is used (Table 1).

1. Prepare 12–15 sections (approximately 90 μm apart) spanning the knee joint for each experimental group. A minimum of ten animals per group per time point (*see* Subheading 3.3.7 for further details).

2. Score the medial tibial plateau and medial femoral condyle of all samples, since damage observed post-DMM surgery is located primarily on the medial side of the joint (*see* Fig. 5 for grading of four quadrants of the knee joint).

3. Repeat scoring by a minimum of two individuals.

4. Represent data as SUM Score (where the summed OA score of a recommended total of ten slides is graphically represented for each mouse/knee) or MAX score (where the maximum score for each mouse/knee is represented graphically) (*see* Fig. 6 for representative sections of each OA grade).

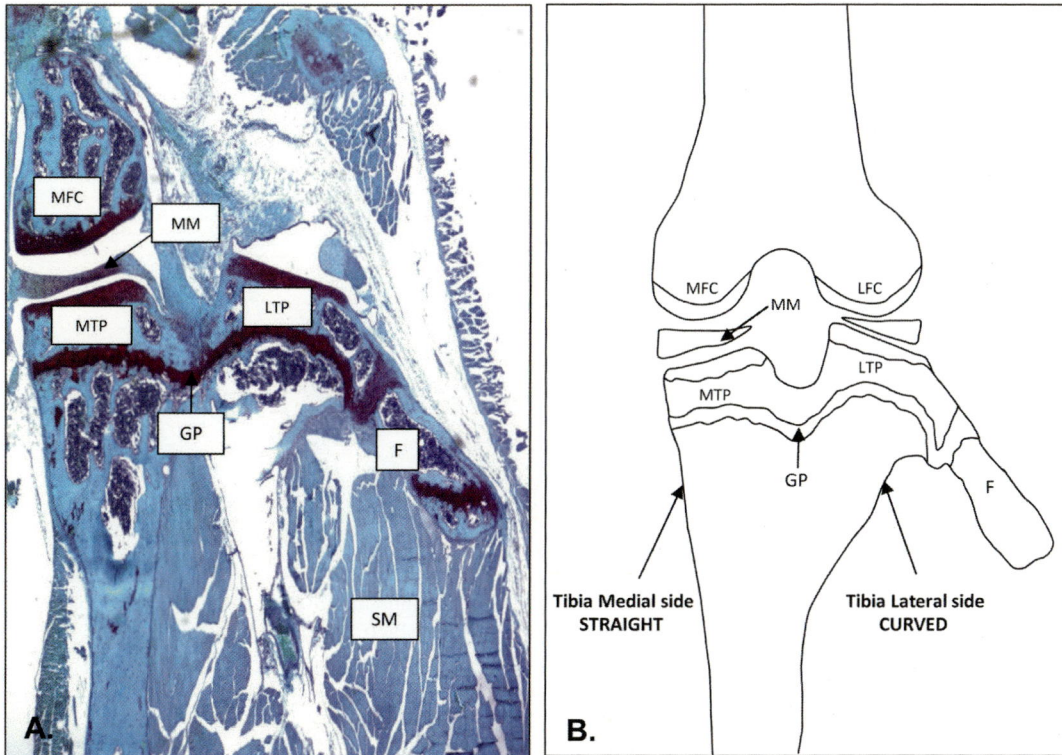

Fig. 4 Representative photomicrograph of Safranin O-stained coronal section (**a**) and schematic (**b**) detailing the anatomical structures of the knee. Three quadrants are visualized: medial femoral condyle (MFC), medial tibial plateau (MTP), and lateral tibial plateau (LTP). The growth plate (GP) is located at the proximal end of tibia (T) and fibula (F). Skeletal muscle, (SM) can be seen surrounding the knee. The medial meniscus (M) can be identified between the MTP and MFC

Table 1
Mouse histological scoring system recommended by OARSI [32]

Grade	Osteoarthritis damage
0	Normal
0.5	Loss of Safranin O without structural changes
1	Small fibrillations without loss of cartilage
2	Fibrillation to the layer immediately below the superficial layer and some loss of surface lamina
3	Fibrillation/erosion to the calcified cartilage extending to <25 % of the width of articular cartilage
4	Fibrillation/erosion to the calcified cartilage extending to 25–50 % of the width of articular cartilage
5	Fibrillation/erosion to the calcified cartilage extending to 50–75 % of the width of articular cartilage
6	Fibrillation/erosion to the calcified cartilage extending to >75 % of the width of articular cartilage

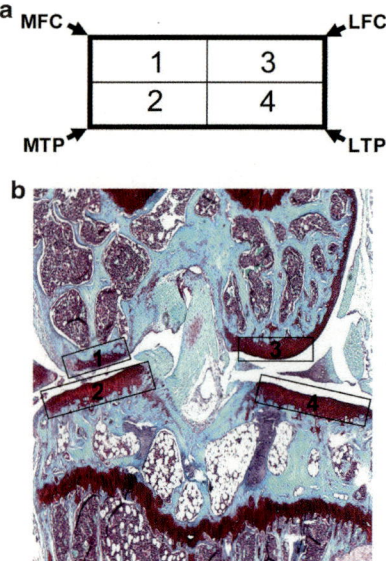

Fig. 5 Schematic (**a**) and Safranin O-stained coronal section. (**b**) Representation of the four quadrants of the knee, which can be graded post-DMM surgery, including the medial tibial plateau (MTP), medial femoral condyle (MFC), lateral tibial plateau (LTP), and lateral femoral condyle (LFC). The majority of cartilage damage will be observed on the medial side of the joint

3.3.7 Statistical Analysis

1. Perform power analysis for the number of mice required per group. Using a 2-point difference as the definition of a statistical difference, group sample sizes of 7 mice in each group achieves 85.8 % power to detect a 2-point difference in the modified mouse score after adjusting for nonparametric Mann-Whitney U test and setting significance to 0.017 (to adjust for multiple comparisons). To account for attrition due to surgery or anesthesia-related deaths, the total number per group is adjusted to 10.

2. For histological scoring, Mann-Whitney U tests and Kruskal-Wallis with Dunn's post-analysis (Prism® Graph-Pad) are needed as the nonparametric equivalents for the independent samples t-test and one-way ANOVA (*see* **Note 13**).

3.3.8 Osteophyte Scoring

The progressive erosion of the cartilage observed post-DMM surgery is accompanied by osteophyte formation and development. The DMM model is a valuable tool to assess the contribution of certain genes to the formation and development of osteophytes during OA. Indeed, Loeser and colleagues [33] described in detail the relationship between osteophyte development in OA and genes involved in morphogenesis, differentiation, and development. A histological scoring system was developed to score both osteophyte size and maturity, as described by Little et al. [15] (*see* Tables 2

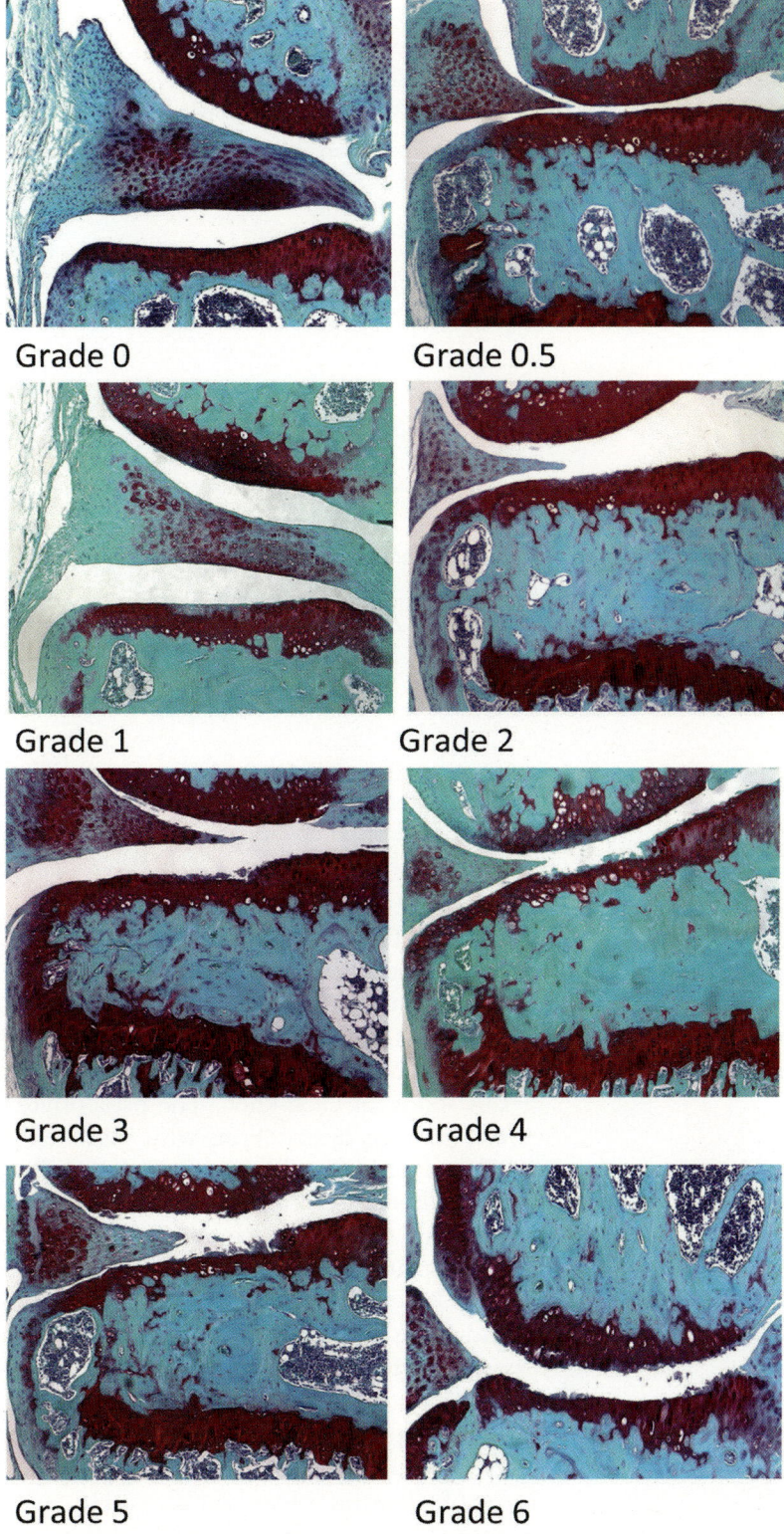

Fig. 6 Safranin O-stained coronal sections taken from the knee representing each OA grade of the modified Mankin scoring system recommended by OARSI [32]. The grade presented represents the damage observed on the medial tibial plateau. Graphs can be constructed based on scoring of multiple knee joints using Table 1.

Table 2
Assessment of osteophyte size in mouse knee joints

Osteophyte size	Features
0	None
1	Small (approx. same thickness as the adjacent cartilage)
2	Medium (approx. 1–3 times the thickness of the adjacent cartilage)
3	Large (approx. >3 times the thickness of the adjacent cartilage)

Table 3
Assessment of osteophyte maturity in mouse knee joints

Osteophyte maturity	Features
0	None
1	Predominantly cartilage
2	Mix of cartilage and bone
3	Predominantly bone

and 3). This system complements the modified Mankin scoring system recommended by OARSI [32] for grading cartilage degradation, and follows the same scoring guidelines for statistical analysis. Briefly, osteophyte scoring is performed on the same slides/sections used to assess cartilage degradation and obtain an OA score for each knee. The osteophyte size is highly dependent on cartilage destruction, with joints exhibiting a high OA score often also having large mature osteophytes (Fig. 7). In addition, osteophytes are often localized close to areas of cartilage degradation, and thus are predominately located on the medial side of the tibial plateau. Initially, osteophytes are composed of cartilage (Fig. 7a, e), and then transition to a combination of both cartilage and bone (b) before they progress to a boney appearance as the osteophyte matures (Fig. 7b, f).

3.4 Immuno-histochemistry

Localization of protein targets of interest, including MMP-13, or the presence of type II collagen cleavage epitopes (C1,2C) are examined by immunohistochemistry (IHC) using commercially available antibodies (e.g., from Abcam, or Ibex http://www.ibex.ca) or in-house generated antibodies, if necessary (*see* **Note 14**). Depending upon the selected antibody or the tissue processing (fixation, decalcification method, etc.), the optimal antigen retrieval method, the primary and secondary antibody concentration, or the antibody

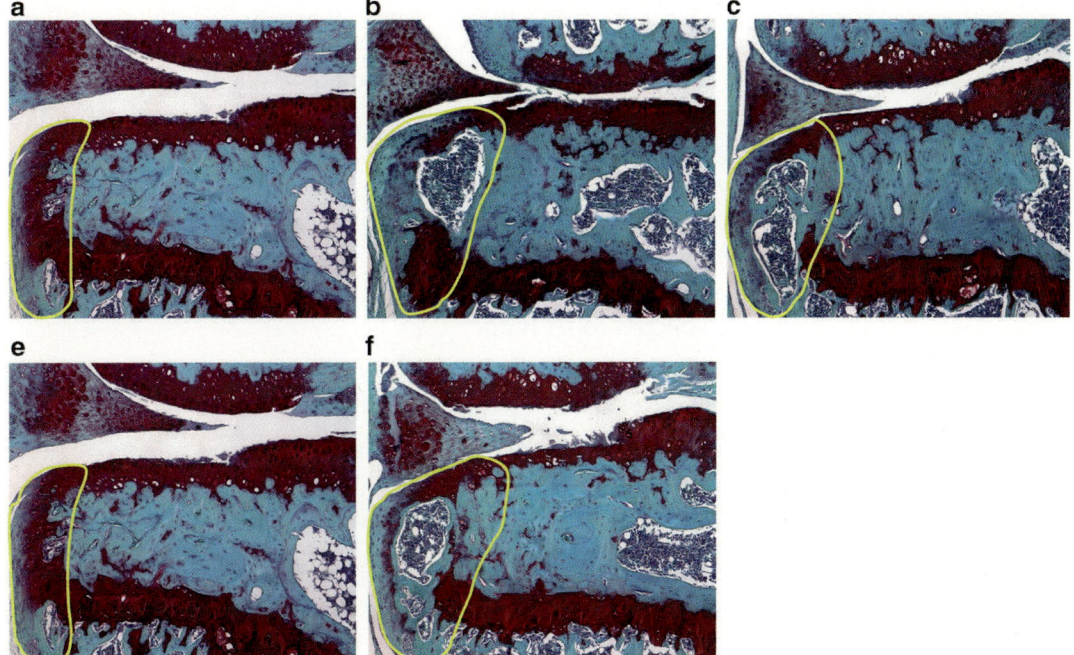

Fig. 7 Representative photomicrograph images of Safranin O-stained coronal sections taken from the knee (wild-type mouse post-DMM surgery) with *yellow outlines* indicating osteophytes. The composition of the osteophyte is dependent on its maturity: Early osteophytes are composed mainly of cartilage (**a**), and then transition to a combination of both cartilage and bone (**b**) before they develop into mature osteophytes that consist mainly of bone (**c**). The size and maturity of the osteophyte often correlates with the severity of OA found in the joint post surgery, with small osteophytes consisting mainly of cartilage observed in joints with a low histological score (**e**), and mature osteophytes consisting mainly of bone observed in highly damaged joints (**f**). Graphs can be constructed based on scoring of multiple knee joints using Tables 2 and 3

blocking solution will vary, and therefore each IHC protocol should be carefully optimized. Below is provided an example of an IHC protocol using the C1,2C antibody (IBEX #50-1035) on formalin-fixed, sodium citrate: formic acid-decalcified, paraffin-embedded knee sections in mice post-DMM.

3.4.1 Immunoperoxidase Staining

1. Deparaffinize sections in xylene, 2× for 10 min each.

2. Rehydrate gradually through a series of graded ethanol concentrations: 100 % (2×, 3 min each); 95 % (2 min); 85 % (1 min); 70 % (1 min); 50 % (1 min). Finally, wash in 1× PBS (2×, 5 min each).

3. Perform antigen retrieval treatment with 2 mg/mL hyaluronidase for 30 min at 37 °C in a humid chamber (*see* **Note 15**).

4. Wash in 1× PBS buffer (3× for 5 min).

5. Incubate for 15 min at RT in 3 % hydrogen peroxide in dH$_2$O to quench endogenous peroxidase activity.

6. Wash in 1× PBS buffer (2× for 5 min).

7. Incubate in 1.5 % normal goat blocking solution in a humid chamber for at least 1 h at room temperature (*see* **Note 16**).

8. Remove blocking solution from slides and incubate with primary antibody C1,2C at 1: 200 dilution or the corresponding isotype-matched negative control (*see* **Note 17**) in the normal goat blocking buffer with 1.5 % Tween overnight at 4 °C in a humid chamber.

9. Wash in 1× PBS buffer (2× for 5 min). Optional: Add 0.5 % Tween to the 1× PBS buffer from this step if the background is expected to be high.

10. Incubate with biotin-conjugated secondary antibody for 1 h at room temperature in a humid chamber.

11. Wash in 1× PBS buffer (2× for 5 min).

12. Incubate with avidin biotin enzyme reagent for 30 min at room chamber in a humid chamber.

13. Wash in 1× PBS buffer (2× for 5 min).

14. Incubate with DAB chromogen or Vector NovaRed until desired stain intensity develops. Comparative slides (e.g., wild-type versus knockout and positive and negative controls) should be monitored to determine the proper development time.

15. Wash sections in dH_2O for 2 min to stop the reaction.

16. The provided C1,2C IHC protocol does not include a counterstaining step. If required, counterstaining methods include:

    (a) Fast green 0.2 % solution: stain for 2 min, followed by quick washing in 95 % EtOH.

    (b) Hematoxylin (filtered): Stain for 30 s, followed by immediate washing with several changes of dH_2O, then with 95 % EtOH.

17. Rinse quickly in 100 % EtOH, and then perform a second wash in 100 % EtOH for 2 min.

18. Incubate in Xylene (2× for 5 min).

19. Mount slides with two drops of Vectamount medium, cover with a glass coverslip, and observe by light microscopy.

3.4.2 Immunofluorescence Staining Protocol

The immunofluorescence (IF) protocol is commonly used when there is a need to detect multiple cellular targets by simultaneous labeling; a mix of primary antibodies is followed by a combination of secondary antibodies conjugated to diverse fluorochromes emitting light at different wavelengths. The following protocol is intended as a general guide for immunofluorescence on paraffin embedded sections:

1. Follow **steps 1–4** of the IHC protocol (Subheading 3.4.1).

2. Incubate with normal blocking serum for 1 h at room temperature in a humid chamber (*see* **Note 16**).

3. Incubate with optimized primary antibody concentration in a humid chamber overnight at 4 °C (*see* **Note 17**). If using a primary antibody conjugated with a fluorochrome, omit **step 5**.

4. Wash in 1× PBS buffer with 0.05 % Tween 20 (2× for 5 min).

5. Incubate with fluorochrome-conjugated secondary antibody for 1–2 h at room temperature in a humid chamber (make sure from this step onwards the samples are shielded from light). Secondary antibodies are conjugated to a wide range of fluorochromes to suit the users needs (e.g., IgG-FITC, IgG-TR, IgG-CY3, IgG-Cy5, Alexa Fluor or DyLight, Chromeo, and SureLight). As cartilage auto fluoresces in the green spectrum it is recommended to use fluorochromes that do not fall within this spectrum.

6. Wash in 1× PBS buffer with 0.05 % Tween 20 (2× for 5 min) in a slide container covered with aluminum foil.

7. Mount slides with an antifade mounting medium (e.g., ProLong Gold antifade reagent with DAPI) and follow drying instructions of the manufacturer.

8. Visualize staining with a fluorescence microscope.

3.5 RNA Extraction for Gene Expression Analysis

For RNA isolation, cartilage is dissected from the femoral heads and tibial plateaus of the knee and homogenized in TRIzol. The total RNA is isolated using the *mir*Vana miRNA isolation kit following the manufacturer's instructions with additional modifications. Following this method, an average of 50–125 ng of total RNA is obtained from the articular cartilage isolated from one knee joint. This should serve as a guide as to how many mice are required to achieve a required amount of RNA for gene expression analyses.

It is critical to place each leg in RNAlater (**steps 1–5**) as early as possible to obtain good RNA integrity; thus, one person completes **steps 1–7** and a second person completes **steps 8–12**.

Person 1:

1. Sacrifice mouse and immediately remove hind legs.

2. Use dissection scissors to remove as much soft tissue from the legs as possible.

3. Place the legs in separate Petri dishes and cover with ice-cold 1× PBS.

4. While working on one leg, keep the other leg in 1× PBS on ice, complete **steps 5–7** on the other leg.

5. Dissect remaining muscle and tendon with a scalpel and size 15 blade under the microscope. Remove dissected soft tissues from the Petri dish, as these tissues may be sources of RNases.

6. Transfer cleaned leg to a fresh Petri dish and wash with ice-cold 1× PBS.

7. Transfer the washed leg into a fresh small Petri dish and cover with RNAlater. Keep the leg on ice in RNAlater until ready to complete **steps 8–13**.

   Person 2: Keep legs in RNAlater at all times during the following steps in the Petri dish placed under the dissection microscope, use a scalpel with size 11 blade to separate the tibia and femur and expose the articular surfaces.

8. Remove any remaining soft tissue or tendon surrounding the articular surfaces with a scalpel or small dissection scissors. Be careful not to damage the cartilage.

9. Place the bones in a fresh Petri dish and cover with RNA later, as small amounts of soft tissue will make dissected cartilage difficult to decipher.

10. While the leg is bathed in RNAlater use a scalpel with size 11 blade to carve the cartilage from the articular surfaces of the tibia and femur.

11. Place the harvested cartilage in RNase free Eppendorf tube containing RNAlater (enough to completely cover the cartilage sample). Samples can be pooled in order to obtain a higher RNA yield.

12. Either:

    (a) Proceed immediately with the RNA isolation using the *mir*Vana kit and the modified protocol below; or

    (b) Place the cartilage in RNAlater overnight at 4 °C. Remove excess RNA later in the morning, and store at −80 °C until ready to isolate RNA.

3.6 RNA Isolation from Cartilage Using Modified mirVana miRNA Isolation Kit (Ambion) Protocol

The following procedure is performed according to the manufacturer's instructions (*see* **Note 18**), except that additional phenol; chloroform steps have been introduced to help improve the 260/280 values of the RNA isolated. To obtain good RNA integrity (RIN) values, all reagents, pipet tips and Eppendorf tubes must be certified nuclease-free. In addition, isolation should be completed on a clean work space treated with RNAse Zap (Ambion).

1. Place the Eppendorf tube containing cartilage sample on ice and add 500 µL of TRIzol to the tube. Homogenize the cartilage sample in TRIzol using a 1.5-mL RNAse-free pestle and hand-held homogenizer, for approximately 5–10 min. Each knee can be homogenized separately, with the option of pooling multiple samples onto the *mir*Vana filter column at **step 19**.

2. Add 200 µL TRIzol (to total volume of 700 µL) and vortex to mix.

3. Transfer TRIzol with disrupted tissue to QIAshredder to further homogenize and disrupt cells: centrifuge 2 min at $16,000 \times g$.

4. Transfer sample to a fresh nuclease-free Eppendorf tube, taking care not to take or disrupt the pellet of matrix that will be visible.

5. Add 300 µL TRIzol and vortex to mix (total volume: 1 mL).

6. Add 200 µL chloroform:IAA per 1 mL TRIzol and vortex for 15 s.

7. Incubate samples on ice for 5 min.

8. Centrifuge at $13,000 \times g$ for 10 min at 4 °C.

9. Remove the aqueous phase, taking care not to disrupt the interface, and transfer to new RNase-free tube (make note of volume).

10. Add 1 volume of phenol:chloroform:IAA to the aqueous phase and vortex for 15 s.

11. Incubate on ice for 10 min.

12. Centrifuge for at $16,000 \times g$ for 15 min at 4 °C.

13. Remove aqueous phase and transfer to new RNase free tube (make note of volume).

14. Add 1 volume of chloroform:IAA to the aqueous phase, vortex 15 s to mix.

15. Incubate on ice for 5 min.

16. Centrifuge at $9,300 \times g$, 10 min, 4 °C.

17. Remove aqueous phase and transfer to new RNase-free tube (make note of volume).

18. Add 1.25× aqueous volume of nuclease-free 100 % ethanol (room temperature) to the aqueous phase.

    From this step onwards, reagents from the *mir*Vana miRNA isolation kit will be used. These steps will isolate total RNA, including miRNA, within the same fraction. However, the kit also provides the option for isolating miRNA and mRNA in different fractions (refer to the user's manual included with the kit for further information).

19. For each sample, place a *mir*Vana filter cartridge into a collection tube. Add the lysate/ethanol mix to the filter, 700 µL at a time, and centrifuge (~15 s, $10,000 \times g$, room temperature). Discard flow through. (For sample volumes larger than 700 µL repeat in successive applications to the same filter.)

20. Apply 700 µL of miRNA wash solution 1 (*mir*Vana Kit) to column and centrifuge (~5 to 10 s, $10,000 \times g$, room temperature). Discard flow-through.

21. Apply 500 μL of miRNA wash solution 2/3 (*mir*Vana Kit) to column and centrifuge (~5 to 10 s, 10,000×*g*, RT). Discard flow-through.

22. Repeat **step 21**.

23. Spin column to remove residual fluid (1 min, 10,000×*g*, room temperature).

24. Transfer filter cartridge to fresh collection tube.

25. Add 100–50 μL nuclease-free water (room temperature) to the filter and leave for 1 min.

26. Centrifuge to elute (~30 s, 16,000×*g*) (*see* **Note 19**).

27. Apply the eluted sample to the filter cartridge and spin again (~30 s, 16,000×*g*) (*see* **Note 20**).

28. To a 50 μL-volume of RNA, sample add 0.1 volume (5 μL) of DNase buffer and 1 μL DNase (all reagents provided with the DNA-free Kit from Ambion).

29. Incubate at 37 °C for 25 min.

30. Add 0.1 volume (5.5 μL) of inactivating reagent, mix well, and incubate at room temperature for 2 min (mixing occasionally, at least three times).

31. Centrifuge at 10,000×*g*, 1.5 min, 4 °C.

32. Remove the supernatant and place in a nuclease-free 1.5-mL tube.

33. Quantify RNA using a NanoDrop spectrophotometer.

34. RNA integrity value can be assessed at this point using a Bioanalyzer through a service usually provided by the institutional genomics core.

Ethanol Precipitation

This precipitation step can be completed to concentrate the RNA if the concentration obtained above is not enough for required analyses.

1. On ice, add 94 μL of ice-cold water to each 50 μL of RNA sample (volumes should now be about 144 μL).

2. Add 16 μL of cold 3 M NaOAc, pH 5.0, to each sample to make a concentration of around 0.3 M. Mix by pipetting up and down. Final volume will be 160 μL.

3. To each sample add 2 μL of 20 μg/μL UltraPure Glycogen (*see* **Note 21**).

4. Add 2.5 parts of ice-cold 100 % ethanol to each sample—pipette up and down to mix.

5. Place the samples at –80 °C for at least 1 h (can be left overnight).

6. Centrifuge at maximum speed, 10 min at 4 °C.

7. The RNA pellet should now be visible in the Eppendorf tube. Decant ethanol.

8. Add 750 μL of ice-cold 70 % ethanol to the pellet, gently vortex, and centrifuge at $10,000 \times g$ for 5 min.

9. The RNA pellet should now be visible. Decant ethanol. Centrifuge samples quickly (approximately 5 s) to collect any remaining ethanol in the bottom of the tube and remove it with a filtered, nuclease-free tip.

10. Resuspend RNA in 10–15 μL of sterile nuclease-free water.

11. Re-assess RNA concentration using a NanoDrop spectrophotometer.

12. Assess RIN value using a Bioanalyzer.

---

4 Notes

1. To induce Cre-recombinase-mediated deletion of the floxed gene only in adult chondrocytes, mice receive three intraperitoneal injections of either tamoxifen (knockout) or vehicle alone (wild-type control) at 2-day intervals of 2.0 mg per 10 g of body weight of mouse. However, the concentration and dose should be chosen carefully depending on the age of the animal, and therefore the current literature should be reviewed. The final injection is scheduled 1 week prior to surgery, which is usually performed at 12 weeks of age, allowing the mice time for complete gene ablation and recovery from tamoxifen treatment before anesthesia. To observe the effects of gene modification on OA development, comparisons should be done in tamoxifen- versus vehicle-treated littermates.

2. Different doxycycline concentrations have been used successfully, with no reported adverse effects [28, 29], but with differences in the time required for transgene activation to occur due to the varying amount of time required for doxycycline to clear from the mouse system. The concentrations achieved by the doses administered are not sufficient to inhibit collagenase activity. Adequate controls have to be used for comparison after the DMM surgery [29].

3. All procedures must be approved by the Institutional Animal Care and Use Committee (IACUC). Before live animals are used, all personnel must obtain CLAS orientation and training, including demonstration to veterinarians the surgical procedure on cadaveric mice.

4. *See* Glasson et al. [30] for excellent photographs and schematics to guide the surgery.

5. It is recommended that one surgeon perform all surgeries involving each genetically modified mouse strain to reduce variability. Comparisons between wild-type and knockout or transgenic strains are completed using littermates. Nonoperated or sham controls need to be checked to ensure that there is no nonspecific effect of the genetic modification.

6. The fat pad may also be left in place and merely transected to allow access and visualization of the MMTL, although this may significantly affect the outcome of the DMM surgery.

7. Significant postoperative pain and debility are not anticipated. Mice are monitored postoperatively by the Veterinary Staff, and if there is evidence of pain, suffering or illness, analgesia and/or other treatment will be administered at their discretion. Particular attention will be paid to ensure that animals are ambulating normally after the procedure. For further information on analgesic dugs, please *see* reviews [31, 34].

8. Since only male mice are used in the DMM model because of the protection by estrogen in females [30], it is necessary to establish the following procedures to avoid aggressive behavior. Mice are housed together prior to surgery (completed as soon as possible post weaning if males are not from the same litter), and the same mice are housed together post-surgery. Administration of analgesics is continued according to the protocol. Surgical mice are monitored for the first few hours after surgery and immediately the next morning. If a dominant male is noticed, it is immediately separated from the group. The remaining mice in the cage are monitored daily for fighting and any new emerging dominant male is removed. A minimum of three mice must remain housed together post surgery to encourage the level of activity required to promote OA initiation, development, and progression.

9. Immediately after surgery, place one mouse tunnel per cage to provide enrichment and promote the level of activity required to promote OA initiation, development, and progression.

10. For histology, mice may be sacrificed by CO_2 inhalation. For RNA extraction, if a CO_2 tank is not immediately available, cervical dislocation may be required to avoid rigor mortis before tissues can be dissected from the joints and placed in extraction buffer.

11. Alternatively to test if the samples are decalcified, a needle can be passed through the bone of the sample. If no resistance is felt, the sample can be considered decalcified.

12. During sectioning check carefully to ensure the knee is correctly orientated in the paraffin. The lateral femoral condyle will usually appear in the first sections. Refer to Figs. 4 and 5 to gain a good concept of the proper knee orientation. If the knee is

found to be in the incorrect orientation and all four quadrants are not identified, you can attempt to re-embed the knee in the correct orientation.

13. Previous studies by Glasson et al. [30] found that the mean maximum histological scores at 4 weeks postoperatively for the unoperated, sham surgery, and DMM groups, respectively, were (±S.E.M.) 1.1 ± 0.1, 1.0 ± 0.3, 3.7 ± 1.5 and 4.3 ± 0.4; and at 8 weeks the mean maximum scores were 1.2 ± 0.3, 1.2 ± 0.2, 4.1 ± 0.3, 5.0 ± 0.4.

14. The conditions for immunohistochemistry and immunofluorescence (e.g., antigen retrieval method and primary and secondary antibody concentration) may vary and require optimization. The provided protocols are guidelines, and have been optimized for applying the specified antibodies to mouse knee joints utilizing the reagents indicated.

15. Hyaluronidase treatment is just one of many available antigen retrieval methods. In general, the retrieval method depends upon the antibody selected and the tissue processing, and therefore requires optimization for the antibody used for detection of specific antigen epitopes in a given tissue. It is advisable to perform optimization steps comparing conditions without antigen retrieval with one or two antigen retrieval methods. Retrieval methods include but are not limited to:

    (a) Heat retrieval in a sodium citrate buffer pH 6.0 (20 min at 95 °C).

    (b) Treatment with hyaluronidase (2 mg/mL 30 min at 37 °C).

    (c) Treatment with pepsin (5 mg/mL in 0.02 % HCl, for 45 min at 37 °C).

    (d) Treatment with 0.05 % saponin solution for 30 min RT.

16. Blocking solutions are used to reduce background and diminish nonspecific staining. Many blocking methods exist and the correct method should be used for your chosen antibody. If normal serum is used for blocking, the correct serum should be chosen to avoid interaction with primary and secondary antibodies, and the tissue being stained. Ideally the serum chosen should be derived from the same species in which the secondary antibody is raised, or from an unrelated species. Increasing the incubation time with blocking serum can further reduce background staining. In addition, adding nonionic detergents (such as Tween) can reduce nonspecific hydrophobic interactions and help permeabilize the tissue to reach intracellular epitopes.

17. Optimal antibody concentrations should be determined empirically, by titration in the blocking buffer. Always incubate slides with positive (tissue known to express your protein of interest control or commercially available positive controls) and negative

controls (isotype nonimmune immunoglobulin control at the same concentration as the primary antibody, or a tissue that does not express the antigen).

18. The *mir*Vana miRNA isolation kit (Ambion) can be purchased with or without phenol. This protocol is optimized using the *mir*Vana kit *without* phenol, with the addition of TRIzol (Invitrogen).

19. Some downstream sequencing protocols require a minimum amount of RNA at a certain concentration (ng) per μL. The 50 μL elution volume is a smaller volume than that recommended by the manufacturer, but can result in more concentrated RNA, which can sometimes prevent the need to complete ethanol precipitation in order to concentrate the sample.

20. Re-apply the eluted sample back onto the filter to increase both yield and concentration of RNA.

21. Glycogen can interfere with some downstream sequencing methods and should be investigated before use as a carrier.

Acknowledgements

Research related to this topic is supported by National Institutes of Health grants R01-AG-022021 and RC4-AR060546.

References

1. Poulet B, Ulici V, Stone TC et al (2012) Time-series transcriptional profiling yields new perspectives on susceptibility to murine osteoarthritis. Arthritis Rheum 64:3256–3266

2. Poulet B, Hamilton RW, Shefelbine S et al (2011) Characterizing a novel and adjustable noninvasive murine joint loading model. Arthritis Rheum 63:137–147

3. Ko FC, Dragomir C, Plumb DA et al (2013) In vivo cyclic compression causes cartilage degeneration and subchondral bone changes in mouse tibiae. Arthritis Rheum 65:1569–1578

4. Sato T, Konomi K, Yamasaki S et al (2006) Comparative analysis of gene expression profiles in intact and damaged regions of human osteoarthritic cartilage. Arthritis Rheum 54:808–817

5. Aigner T, Fundel K, Saas J et al (2006) Large-scale gene expression profiling reveals major pathogenetic pathways of cartilage degeneration in osteoarthritis. Arthritis Rheum 54:3533–3544

6. Glasson SS (2007) In vivo osteoarthritis target validation utilizing genetically-modified mice. Curr Drug Targets 8:367–376

7. Little CB, Fosang AJ (2010) Is cartilage matrix breakdown an appropriate therapeutic target in osteoarthritis–insights from studies of aggrecan and collagen proteolysis? Curr Drug Targets 11:561–575

8. Bernardo BC, Belluoccio D, Rowley L et al (2011) Cartilage intermediate layer protein 2 (CILP-2) is expressed in articular and meniscal cartilage and down-regulated in experimental osteoarthritis. J Biol Chem 286:37758–37767

9. Yasuhara R, Ohta Y, Yuasa T et al (2011) Roles of beta-catenin signaling in phenotypic expression and proliferation of articular cartilage superficial zone cells. Lab Invest 91:1739–1752

10. Lodewyckx L, Cailotto F, Thysen S et al (2012) Tight regulation of wingless-type signaling in the articular cartilage - subchondral bone biomechanical unit: transcriptomics in Frzb-knockout mice. Arthritis Res Ther 14:R16

11. Loeser RF, Olex AL, McNulty MA et al (2012) Microarray analysis reveals age-related differences in gene expression during the development of osteoarthritis in mice. Arthritis Rheum 64:705–717

12. Nuka S, Zhou W, Henry SP et al (2010) Phenotypic characterization of epiphycan-deficient and epiphycan/biglycan double-deficient mice. Osteoarthritis Cartilage 18: 88–96

13. Glasson SS, Askew R, Sheppard B et al (2005) Deletion of active ADAMTS5 prevents cartilage degradation in a murine model of osteoarthritis. Nature 434:644–648

14. Stanton H, Rogerson FM, East CJ et al (2005) ADAMTS5 is the major aggrecanase in mouse cartilage in vivo and in vitro. Nature 434: 648–652

15. Little CB, Barai A, Burkhardt D et al (2009) Matrix metalloproteinase 13-deficient mice are resistant to osteoarthritic cartilage erosion but not chondrocyte hypertrophy or osteophyte development. Arthritis Rheum 60:3723–3733

16. Echtermeyer F, Bertrand J, Dreier R et al (2009) Syndecan-4 regulates ADAMTS-5 activation and cartilage breakdown in osteoarthritis. Nat Med 15:1072–1076

17. Lin AC, Seeto BL, Bartoszko JM et al (2009) Modulating hedgehog signaling can attenuate the severity of osteoarthritis. Nat Med 15: 1421–1425

18. Sampson ER, Hilton MJ, Tian Y et al (2011) Teriparatide as a chondroregenerative therapy for injury-induced osteoarthritis. Sci Transl Med 3:101ra193

19. Chockalingam PS, Sun W, Rivera-Bermudez MA et al (2011) Elevated aggrecanase activity in a rat model of joint injury is attenuated by an aggrecanase specific inhibitor. Osteoarthritis Cartilage 19:315–323

20. Johnson K, Zhu S, Tremblay MS et al (2012) A stem cell-based approach to cartilage repair. Science 336:717–721

21. Rai MF, Hashimoto S, Johnson EE et al (2012) Heritability of articular cartilage regeneration and its association with ear-wound healing. Arthritis Rheum 64:2300–2310

22. Hashimoto S, Rai MF, Janiszak KL et al (2012) Cartilage and bone changes during development of post-traumatic osteoarthritis in selected LGXSM recombinant inbred mice. Osteoarthritis Cartilage 20:562–571

23. Nakamura E, Nguyen MT, Mackem S (2006) Kinetics of tamoxifen-regulated Cre activity in mice using a cartilage-specific CreER(T) to assay temporal activity windows along the proximodistal limb skeleton. Dev Dyn 235: 2603–2612

24. Dao DY, Jonason JH, Zhang Y et al (2012) Cartilage-specific beta-catenin signaling regulates chondrocyte maturation, generation of ossification centers, and perichondrial bone formation during skeletal development. J Bone Miner Res 27:1680–1694

25. Henry SP, Jang CW, Deng JM et al (2009) Generation of aggrecan-CreERT2 knockin mice for inducible Cre activity in adult cartilage. Genesis 47:805–814

26. Henry SP, Liang S, Akdemir KC et al (2012) The postnatal role of Sox9 in cartilage. J Bone Miner Res 27:2511–2525

27. Gossen M, Bujard H (1992) Tight control of gene expression in mammalian cells by tetracycline-responsive promoters. Proc Natl Acad Sci U S A 89:5547–5551

28. Grover J, Roughley PJ (2006) Generation of a transgenic mouse in which Cre recombinase is expressed under control of the type II collagen promoter and doxycycline administration. Matrix Biol 25:158–165

29. Xu L, Polur I, Servais JM et al (2011) Intact pericellular matrix of articular cartilage is required for unactivated discoidin domain receptor 2 in the mouse model. Am J Pathol 179:1338–1346

30. Glasson SS, Blanchet TJ, Morris EA (2007) The surgical destabilization of the medial meniscus (DMM) model of osteoarthritis in the 129/SvEv mouse. Osteoarthritis Cartilage 15:1061–1069

31. Flecknell PA (1996) Laboratory animal anesthesia. Academic, London

32. Glasson SS, Chambers MG, Van Den Berg WB et al (2010) The OARSI histopathology initiative—recommendations for histological assessments of osteoarthritis in the mouse. Osteoarthritis Cartilage 18(Suppl 3):S17–S23

33. Loeser RF, Olex AL, McNulty MA et al (2013) Disease progression and phasic changes in gene expression in a mouse model of osteoarthritis. PLoS One 8:e54633

34. Jenkins WL (1987) Pharmacologic aspects of analgesic drugs in animals: an overview. J Am Vet Med Assoc 191:1231–1240

Chapter 13

Assessment of Knee Joint Pain in Experimental Rodent Models of Osteoarthritis

Margaret J. Piel, Jeffrey S. Kroin, and Hee-Jeong Im

Abstract

Pain assessment in animal models of osteoarthritis is integral to interpretation of a model's utility in representing the clinical condition, and enabling accurate translational medicine. Here we describe two methods for behavioral pain assessments available for use in animal models of experimental osteoarthritic pain: Von Frey filaments and spontaneous activity monitoring.

Key words Pain, Animal models, Rats, Mice, Rodents, Methods, Osteoarthritis, Assessment, Von Frey, Spontaneous activity

1 Introduction

Animal models of osteoarthritis (OA) include those that develop spontaneously or are surgically or nonsurgically (chemically) induced, all of which can provide insights into the molecular, pathological, or biochemical progression of changes in the joint during OA. Chronic pain is a hallmark of OA, and its evaluation in any animal model is integral to assessing the relevance and utility of that model in translation research.

Small animals (primarily mice and rats but also rabbits and guinea pigs) are used extensively in OA research, and a large repository of historical data, especially in rats and mice, exists to which research data can be compared. Their small size and typically lower cost for purchase and maintenance compared with large animals make them attractive animals in which to model OA. Some small animals, such as mice, can be genetically altered to enable the study of specific modulators in the development of OA, and while others, such as the Dunkin Hartley guinea pig, can spontaneously develop OA.

Osteoarthritis pain is typically localized and related to movement or weight-bearing of the affected joint(s), which in animal models are typically the knee and/or hip joint. Pain is difficult to

Jennifer J. Westendorf and Andre J. van Wijnen (eds.), *Osteoporosis and Osteoarthritis*, Methods in Molecular Biology, vol. 1226, DOI 10.1007/978-1-4939-1619-1_13, © Springer Science+Business Media New York 2015

evaluate objectively in humans because of the inherent variability in the individual's interpretation of the sensory input. This variability represents the emotional and cognitive components of pain perception. In addition, little correlation exists between the objective measures of OA (e.g., radiologic or pathologic changes) and the degree of chronic pain experienced by the individual.

Methods used to assess pain in rodents include those that are mechanically, anatomically, or chemically based. The most critical part in any testing method is to ensure that the animal is calm and relaxed before the testing. Many assessments of pain in OA animal models are behaviorally based, and may require that the animals be acclimatized to any apparatus before testing. These behavioral animal tests can usually be carried out at room temperature. Measures for assessing pain in animals can be direct or indirect. Indirect measures include static or dynamic weight-bearing, foot posture, gait analysis, and spontaneous movement. Direct measures include hind limb withdrawal test to mechanical/thermal/cold stimulation, knee compression force, struggle threshold angle of knee extension, knee tissue edema, vocalizations after stimulation of the affected knee, and brain imaging. Here, we describe two methods for the measurement of pain that can be used for experimental OA models in rodents: mechanical sensitivity by use of Von Frey filaments and spontaneous activity.

2 Materials

2.1 Mechanical Sensitivity

1. Von Frey filaments: We will describe the force units in grams, but the units written on the handles of the calibrated Von Frey filaments are in log units.
2. Stainless steel instrument tray stand with grid support.
3. Clear plastic rodent cage.
4. Timer.

2.2 Assessment of Spontaneous Behavior

1. Photobeam activity system to measure open-field activity.
2. Laboratory Animal Behavior Observation Registration and Analysis System (LABORAS, Metris, The Netherlands) for behavior pattern recognition.
3. Scale (with chamber and lid) to measure body weight.

3 Methods

3.1 Von Frey Filaments

1. Place a wire mesh (*see* **Note 1**) across the top of a stainless steel instrument tray holder, from which the solid tray has been removed. Many animal facilities already have such meshes (at least for rats) as part of their standard animal caging.

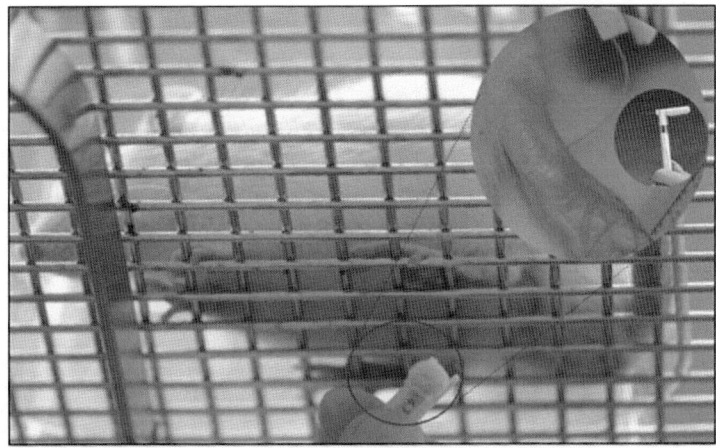

Fig. 1 Mechanical allodynia (Von Frey filament testing). Photograph from below showing rat resting on wire platform and Von Frey filament testing of rat's hind paw. *Inset* shows close-up of filament bending against plantar surface of rat's paw. *Inset within inset* shows close-up of Von Frey filament apparatus

2. Place the rat or mouse on top of the wire mesh, and place the clear plastic rodent cage over the animal (*see* **Note 2**).

3. Allow the animal to explore its surroundings and acclimatize to the test area (*see* **Note 3**).

4. Collect your set of calibrated Von Frey filaments [0.028–5.5 g for mice (2.44–4.74 log units); 0.41–15 g for rats (3.61–5.18 log units)].

5. After 10–15 min, once exploratory behavior has ceased, begin the testing. Using an intermediated value of Von Frey hair [0.4 g in mice (3.61 log unit), 2.0 g in rats (4.31 log unit)], touch the tip of the filament at a right angle to the bottom (midplantar) surface of the rodent's hind foot through the mesh floor until the filament bends. Continued advancement produces more bending but not more force (Fig. 1) (*see* **Note 4**).

6. Wait for at least 5 s, record the response [foot withdrawal (mark X) or no foot withdrawal (mark 0)], and then repeat, using the next higher successive Von Frey filament if there was no response to the previous filament, or the next lower successive Von Frey filament if there was a response to the previous filament.

7. Continue testing until four stimuli have been applied following the first response reversal [i.e., a change from foot withdrawal to no foot withdrawal (X to 0), or, a change from no foot withdrawal to foot withdrawal 0 to X)]. In theory, as many as nine stimuli may be required. If no filament in the set produces any withdrawal then use the default values of 0.02 g in mice and 0.3 g in rats; if all filaments in the set produce withdrawal then use the default values of 6 g in mice and 15 g in rats.

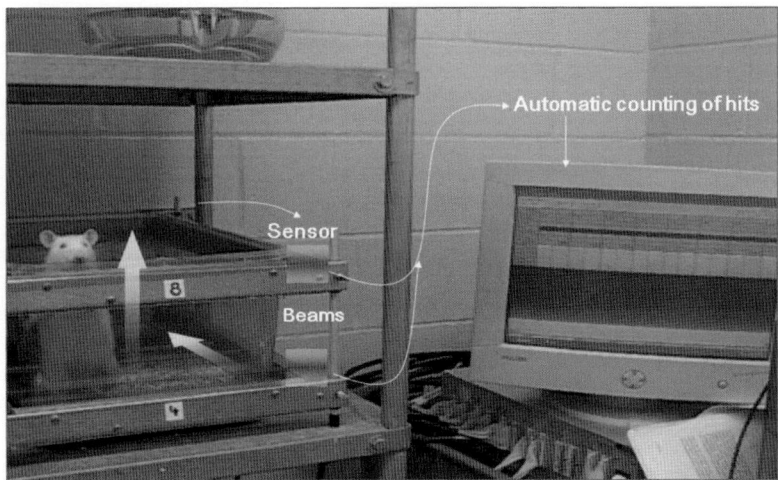

Fig. 2 Spontaneous photobeam activity system for rearing (vertical photobeam crossings) and ambulatory movement (horizontal photobeam crossings)

8. Calculate the threshold force corresponding to 50 % withdrawal using the above up-down iterative method [1, 2].
   The equation for rats is
   Force threshold $(g) = (10^{[\text{last filament value used in log units}+0.244k]}/10^4$,
   where k is obtained from the pattern of Xs and 0s (using the table in Appendix 1 of ref. 1).
   The equation for mice is
   Force threshold $(g) = (10^{[\text{last filament value used in log units}+0.383k]}/10^4$,
   where k is obtained from the pattern of Xs and 0s (using the table in Appendix 1 of ref. 1).

3.2 Photobeam Activity System: Open-Field System

1. Adjust the upper set of photobeams to 5 cm above ground for testing mice and 11 cm for testing rats (*see* **Note 5**).
2. Place the animal within the testing chamber with only a minimal amount of bedding (*see* **Note 6**).
3. Run the software package to monitor open-field activity for rearing (vertical photobeam crossings) and ambulatory activity (horizontal photobeam crossings) (Fig. 2) (*see* **Note 7**).

3.3 Behavior Pattern Recognition: LABORAS

1. Weigh the animal. Enter this datum into the LABORAS system (*see* **Note 8**).
2. Place the animal within the rodent cage portion of the LABORAS system.
3. Start data acquisition.

4 Notes

1. Ensure that the wire mesh surface used for the testing is consistent between all testing sessions. The threshold for pain withdrawal can be influenced by the surface on which the rodents are placed [3]. Sanitize the wire mesh and shoebox cage between animals so that olfactory signals do not distract the animal from becoming quickly acclimated. On any day, use a different set of wire meshes for male versus female rodents to reduce distracting olfactory signals.

2. Placing a clear plastic shoebox-like cage over the animal serves to contain it within the testing area and prevents it from escaping or from falling off the surface. In addition, it is easy to visualize the animal throughout the testing period.

3. Ensure that the room in which the testing is occurring is quiet, warm, and environmentally stable. Sudden unexpected noises can startle animals and affect reliability or reproducibility of test results. Similarly, changes in room temperature can adversely affect the animal's ability to acclimatize to the testing area. Von Frey filaments are composed of nylon plastic, which can be adversely affected by heat and humidity and lose calibration. Newer type filaments can be found made of optical glass fibers, which may obviate these potential problems [4].

4. To minimize observer bias and improve reproducibility, one individual should be responsible for testing all animals. Alternatively, an automated system can be employed. Use of automated systems may be more reliable in evaluating pain in rodents in some circumstances [5]. An electronic Von Frey apparatus (Ugo Basile, Italy) can automatically record the animal's response to user-controlled application of force rate. A touch stimulator transducer is placed on the midplantar surface of the rodent's hind foot, until the foot is lifted by the animal. A display then gives the operator a summary of the results of the force and time corresponding to the response. Software helps in consistent application of force at the desired rate. A dynamic plantar aesthesiometer (Ugo Basile, Italy) is an automated system that allows measurement of the sensitivity threshold in one test with high repetitiveness. It typically consists of a moveable touch-simulator unit, a framed metal mesh, an animal enclosure, and a microprocessor-controlled electronic unit. The animal moves freely within the enclosure positioned on the metal mesh. After the animal has acclimatized to the apparatus and stopped any exploratory behavior, the operator places the touch simulator below the animal's paw. The unit then automatically raises the filament at a

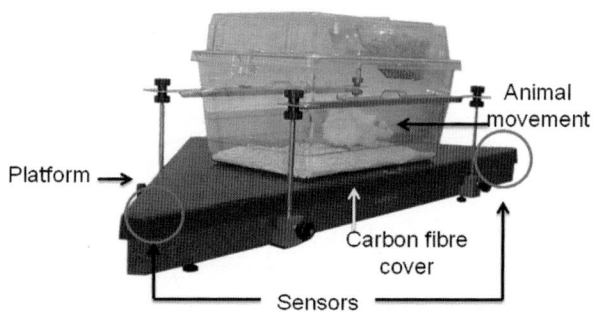

Fig. 3 Spontaneous behavior pattern recognition system by LABORAS. Vibration made by the rat is measured by ultrasensitive sensors located in two corners of the triangular platform

preset force until a signal is received that the animal has either moved its paw or the greatest preset force has been met. Latency to paw withdrawal and force exerted are recorded.

5. Adjacent beams at any height used are 5 cm apart and beam interruptions are recorded automatically. One set of photobeams is set at foot level to measure ambulation (i.e., movement from one beam to another), and an upper set of photobeams is adjusted above ground to measure rearing (i.e., beam breaks in the vertical direction).

6. Activity is monitored in a low-lit room for a predetermined time, typically 60 min. The animal should not be acclimatized to the chamber, since spontaneous exploratory behavior (e.g., rearing) will lessen given prior exposure to the new environment.

7. Photobeam crossings will be recorded automatically. It is best if the investigator leaves the room. Rearing may be affected by the presence of OA.

8. The animal must be accurately weighed before each session. Once the body weight is entered into the software program, the machine automatically calibrates the system. The LABORAS measures behavior based on analysis of vibration and force signals picked up by sensors in the platform on which the cage is placed (Fig. 3). Pattern recognition software then determines and quantifies behaviors that may have been changed by OA-induced pain, including hind limb licking, scratching, wet dog shakes, head shakes, head twitches, purposeless chewing, grooming, locomotion, climbing, immobility, and feeding. Position tracking information is also monitored and quantified, including position (X, Y) and position distribution, speed, and traveled distance. Changed behavioral parameters in an experimental OA model can be interpreted to be knee OA-induced pain response [6, 7].

Acknowledgments

This work was supported by NIH NIAMS R01 grants to HJI from AR053220, AR062136 and VA BLD&R Merit Award.

References

1. Chaplan SR, Bach FW, Pogrel JW et al (1994) Quantitative assessment of tactile allodynia in the rat paw. J Neurosci Methods 53: 55–63

2. Osikowicz M, Mika J, Makuch W et al (2008) Glutamate receptor ligands attenuate allodynia and hyperalgesia and potentiate morphine effects in a mouse model of neuropathic pain. Pain 139:117–126

3. Pitcher GM, Ritchie J, Henry JL (1999) Paw withdrawal threshold in the von Frey hair test is influenced by the surface on which the rat stands. J Neurosci Methods 87: 185–193

4. Fruhstorfer H, Gross W, Selbmann O (2001) Von Frey hairs—new materials for a new design. Eur J Pain 5:341–342

5. Nirogi R, Goura V, Shanmuganathan D et al (2012) Comparison of manual and automated filaments for evaluation of neuropathic pain in rats. J Pharmacol Toxicol Methods 66:8–13

6. Inglis JJ, Notley C, Essex D et al (2007) Collagen-induced arthritis as a model of hyperalgesia: functional and cellular analysis of the analgesic actions of TNF blockade. Arthritis Rheum 56:4015–4023

7. Miller RE, Tran PB, Das R et al (2012) CCR2 chemokine receptor signaling mediates pain in experimental osteoarthritis. Proc Natl Acad Sci U S A 109:20602–20607

Chapter 14

Induction of Fully Stabilized Cortical Bone Defects to Study Intramembranous Bone Regeneration

Meghan E. McGee-Lawrence and David F. Razidlo

Abstract

Bone is a regenerative tissue with an innate ability to self-remodel in response to environmental stimuli and the need to repair damage. Rodent models of fracture healing, and in particular genetic mouse models, can be used to study the contributions of specific molecular switches to skeletal repair, as well as to recreate and exacerbate biological development and repair mechanisms in postnatal skeletons. Here, we describe methodology for producing fully stabilized, single-cortex defects in mouse femurs to study mechanisms of intramembranous bone regeneration.

Key words Intramembranous bone formation, Fracture healing, Stabilized defect repair, Mouse model

1 Introduction

The skeleton is a classic example of regenerative biology, as bone possesses an inherent ability to remodel its structure and composition in response to a need to repair damage, modify architecture, or modulate calcium needs within the body. Repair of skeletal fractures occurs when progenitor cells from the periosteum, intact bone tissue, or bone marrow differentiate into chondrocytes that form cartilage and osteoblasts that form bone [1], where the tissue phenotype developed depends on the mechanical strain environment encountered by cells in the repair site [2–4]. In particular, intramembranous bone, which forms without the need for a preceding cartilage template, is generated within a perfectly stabilized fracture [5]. This result can be achieved with careful external fixation of a transverse femoral or tibial defect [4, 6], which can be used to promote immediate or prolonged healing, the latter of which is applied in the process of distraction osteogenesis [7].

Rigid, externally stabilized fractures, while scientifically useful and most relevant to clinical situations, can be technically challenging to produce. An alternative approach for studying intramembranous bone regeneration mechanisms within the appendicular skeleton is

Jennifer J. Westendorf and Andre J. van Wijnen (eds.), *Osteoporosis and Osteoarthritis*, Methods in Molecular Biology, vol. 1226, DOI 10.1007/978-1-4939-1619-1_14, © Springer Science+Business Media New York 2015

to surgically induce a small void in one bone cortex, leaving the remainder of the bone to rigidly stabilize the defect. This approach allows the researcher to functionally investigate healing processes involving pure bone formation. This method gives insight into bone repair mechanisms, and can also be useful for exacerbating or magnifying developmental skeletal changes that only occur over long time periods. For example, $Axin2^{-/-}$ mice develop high bone mass in the appendicular skeleton due to increased Wnt signaling, but this developmental effect is only apparent at older ages (6–12 months of age) [8]. However, $Axin2^{-/-}$ mice rapidly heal single-cortex femoral defects at a faster rate than wild-type littermates, at least as early as 2–3 months of age [9], indicating that the molecular pathway is active in younger mice and is responsive to stresses that require repair.

2   Materials

2.1 Surgical Tools and Materials

1. Hair clippers or depilatory cream (e.g., Nair® hair remover lotion).
2. Recirculating water warming pad and pump.
3. Povidone-iodine antiseptic solution (10 % topical solution).
4. Stainless steel micro-burr drill bit (Fine Science Tools #19008-07, 0.7 mm diameter).
5. Drill: Variable speed rotary tool (e.g., Dremel) and appropriately sized collet, or suitable alternative.
6. Scalpel (#11 or #15).
7. Dissecting forceps and blunt probe.
8. Sutures (Vicryl 7-0 diameter) or tissue adhesive.
9. Isoflurane vaporizer and anesthesia system.
10. Sterile 0.9 % saline for injection.
11. Buprenorphine (Buprenex for injection: 0.3 mg/mL stock concentration, diluted to 0.02 mg/mL in sterile saline for injection).
12. Acetaminophen (liquid suspension, 160 mg in 5 mL stock concentration, diluted to 1 mg/mL in drinking water).

2.2 Analysis Tools and Materials

1. X-ray system.
2. MicroCT system.
3. 10 % neutral buffered formalin.
4. Graded ethanol (EtOH) solutions, 70–100 %.
5. EDTA solution for decalcification.
   (a) 2.0 L dH_2O.

(b) 140 mL NH$_3$OH (add additional 40 mL later for 180 mL total).

(c) 280 g Ethylenediaminetetraacetic acid (EDTA).

- In a chemical fume hood, slowly dissolve 280 g EDTA and 140 mL NH$_3$OH in 2.0 L dH$_2$O with constant stirring.

- Slowly add the remaining NH$_3$OH to bring pH up to 7.1 (approximately 40 mL, but do not go over pH 7.1).

- Store EDTA solution at room temperature.

6. Paraffin tissue-embedding medium.

7. Xylenes, histological grade.

8. Vacuum oven.

9. Microtome.

10. Safranin O/Fast green staining reagents.

(a) Weigert's working solution: 1:1 combination of "solution A" and "solution B", diluted 1:1 with H$_2$O prior to use.

- Solution A: FeCl stock = 0.25 g Ferric Cl, 15 mL H$_2$O, 0.17 mL concentrated HCl.

- Solution B: Hematoxylin stock = 0.17 g hematoxylin, 1.5 mL 100 % EtOH, diluted in an additional 13.5 mL 95 % EtOH.

(b) 0.001 % Fast green solution (FCF C.I. 42053): 0.25 g fast green, 250 mL H$_2$O.

(c) 0.1 % Safranin O solution (C.I. 50240): 0.1 g safranin O, 100 mL H$_2$O.

(d) 1 % acetic acid solution: 1 mL glacial acetic acid, 99 mL H$_2$O, mixed fresh.

11. Von Kossa silver nitrate/MacNeal's tetrachrome staining reagents.

(a) Silver nitrate solution: 5 g silver nitrate, 100 mL distilled water. Filter before use.

(b) Sodium carbonate-formaldehyde solution: 5 g sodium carbonate, 25 mL formaldehyde, 75 mL distilled water.

(c) Farmer's diminisher: 20 g sodium thiosulfate, 210 mL distilled water. Dissolve sodium thiosulfate in 210 mL distilled water first, and then add 1 g potassium ferricyanide.

- This solution is stable for 45 min once potassium ferricyanide is added. Mix a fresh batch for each use.

(d) MacNeal's tetrachrome: 2 g MacNeal's tetrachrome powder, 100 mL distilled water. Combine and bring briefly to a boil. Remove from heat and stir, at least overnight. Filter before use.

3 Methods

3.1 Prepare Tools and Animal(s) for Surgery

1. Twenty-four hours prior to surgery, begin administration of acetaminophen in the drinking water (1 mg/mL final concentration) for ad libitum consumption (*see* **Note 1**).

2. Sterilize all surgical tools in an autoclave prior to use, and sanitize between animals with a hot bead sterilizer (preferred method) or another acceptable means.

3. One hour prior to surgery, inject animal with buprenorphine (0.1 mg/kg body mass, subcutaneous injection) to provide analgesia.

4. Prepare one hind leg for aseptic surgery by removing hair from the lateral surface of the thigh (shave hair or apply depilatory cream and wash/rinse thoroughly) [10].

5. Induce anesthesia in an isoflurane vaporizer chamber with 3–5 % isoflurane, 3.0 LPM oxygen delivery rate.

6. Transfer mouse to a nose cone and reduce isoflurane administration to 1–2 % concentration for anesthesia maintenance.

7. Place mouse on a recirculating water warming pad to maintain a constant body temperature of 36–38 °C while under anesthesia. Monitor respiration at all times to ensure lack of respiratory distress.

8. Swab skin surface with povidone-iodine antiseptic solution to sanitize immediately prior to surgery.

3.2 Surgical Procedures

1. Create an incision through the skin (but not the underlying muscle) on the lateral surface of the thigh, centered over top of the femur extending roughly along the length of the femoral diaphysis with a #11 or #15 scalpel blade.

2. Expose the femur via blunt dissection with a probe and/or forceps, without transecting muscle tissues.

3. Visually identify anatomical landmarks on the femur including the greater trochanter and the knee joint capsule, and estimate the midpoint between identified landmarks on the anterior surface of the bone. Grip the bone with dissecting forceps immediately above and below the intended defect location, using forceps to retract soft tissues.

4. Create a *single-cortex* drilled defect in the anterior aspect of the bone using a 0.7 mm diameter burr drill bit and a rotary drill speed of approximately 10,000 rpm.

    (a) Irrigate the wound with sterile saline to avoid thermal necrosis and rinse the newly created defect to dislodge any bone fragments.

    (b) Do not continue the defect into or through the opposite cortical bone wall.

5. Immediately after defect creation, obtain an X-ray of the operated leg to ensure proper defect location and the lack of full transverse fracture.

6. Suture the skin incision with 7-0 diameter sutures, or close incision with tissue adhesive.

7. Transfer the animal to a dry, clean cage and ensure recovery from anesthesia (*see* **Note 2**).

8. Administer 0.1 mg/kg buprenorphine subcutaneously at 12 and 24 h after surgery to ensure adequate analgesia, and check wound closure periodically to ensure proper healing.

3.3 Longitudinal Monitoring of Healing via X-Ray

1. Defect healing can be monitored via radiography after surgery. Typical time points include 7, 14, and 21 days after surgery (Fig. 1).

2. Induce anesthesia with isoflurane prior to X-ray as described in Subheading 3.1.

3. Ensure consistent animal positioning to permit longitudinal evaluation of bone defect radiopacity over time. This can be easily done with a radiolucent template to guide animal placement.

4. Perform other procedures (e.g., fluorochrome labeling) as necessary (*see* **Note 3**).

3.4 Tissue Harvest and Storage

1. Sacrifice mouse by carbon dioxide inhalation at postoperative time point of choice. Suggested time points include the following:

   (a) Postoperative day 7: immunohistochemistry, signaling analysis of early healing mechanisms.

   (b) Postoperative day 14 or 21: histology, quantification of bone architecture at mid-healing stages via microCT.

   (c) Postoperative day 28: histology, bone architecture at endpoints of healing via microCT. Wild-type mice regularly demonstrate complete healing by this time point [5],

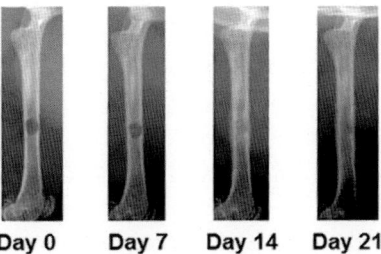

Day 0   Day 7   Day 14   Day 21

Fig. 1 Longitudinal X-ray monitoring of defect repair in a wild-type mouse. Note the increasing radiopacity of the defect over time

and thus this can be a useful time point for comparison of healing in transgenic or mutant mouse strains to wild-type littermates.

2. Remove the operated femur, keeping full bone anatomy intact. Carefully remove overlying soft tissues, but do not disturb tissue makeup in or around the healing defect (*see* **Note 4**).

3. Fix the operated femur in 10 % neutral buffered formalin for 24 h.

4. Transfer to 70 % ethanol for long-term storage.

3.5 Immuno-histochemistry (Decalcified Bone)

1. Remove femoral epiphyses and decalcify femoral diaphysis for at least 7 days in EDTA solution (confirm complete decalcification by X-ray).

2. Dehydrate decalcified tissue through graded ethanols and infiltrate with xylenes and molten paraffin as described below. Note time, temperature, and pressure indicated for each step.

   (a) 70 % EtOH, overnight, room temperature, and pressure (RTP)

   (b) 95 % EtOH, 1.5 h, 60 °C, 15 mmHg vacuum

   (c) 95 % EtOH, 1 h, RTP

   (d) 100 % EtOH, 1.5 h, 60 °C, 15 mmHg vacuum

   (e) 100 % EtOH, 1 h, RTP

   (f) 100 % EtOH, 1 h, RTP

   (g) 100 % EtOH, 1 h, RTP

   (h) Xylenes, 1 h, 60 °C, 15 mmHg vacuum

   (i) Xylenes, 1 h, RTP

   (j) Xylenes, 1 h, RTP

   (k) 50 % Xylenes/50 % molten paraffin, 2 h, 60 °C, 15 mmHg vacuum

   (l) Molten paraffin, 2 h, 60 °C, 15 mmHg vacuum

3. Embed decalcified bone segments in paraffin for longitudinal sectioning; note tissue orientation and location of defect prior to embedding.

4. Obtain longitudinal thin (8 μm) sections through the defect with a microtome.

5. Perform immunohistochemical staining with antibodies of choice according to established protocols [9].

3.6 MicroCT Analysis of Defect Bone Architecture (Undecalcified Bone)

1. Scan the mid-diaphysis of each femur, centered about the defect, in 70 % ethanol with a microCT system at 5–10 μm voxel size. Recommended settings are energy = 70 kVp and integration time = 300 ms.

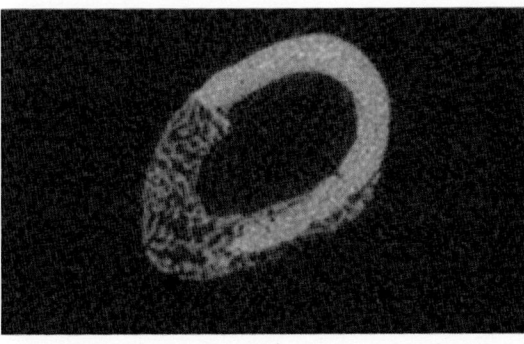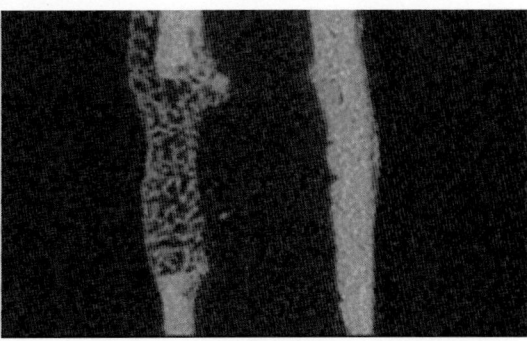

Fig. 2 Transverse and longitudinal images through the center of the defect in a wild-type mouse (postoperative day 14). Images reproduced from ref. 9, with permission

2. Analyze the architecture of the regenerated bone spicules within the defect region (hereafter referred to as "trabecular bone") using the manufacturer's software. Parameters of interest may include bone volume fraction (Tb.BV/TV, %), trabecular number (Tb.N, mm^{-1}), trabecular thickness (Tb.Th, mm), and trabecular separation (Tb.Sp, mm). Report all variables and relevant microCT scan settings according to established guidelines [11].

3. Generate transverse and longitudinal image views from the center of the defect with the manufacturer's software for quantification of defect diameter using image analysis software (Fig. 2).

3.7 Histological Analysis of Tissue Morphology (Decalcified or Undecalcified Bone)

1. Prepare and embed samples via decalcified paraffin embedding (Subheading 3.5) or undecalcified plastic embedding methodology [9, 12, 13] as desired.

2. Obtain thin (5–8 μm) longitudinal bone sections through the center of the healing defect and prepare histologically. Suggested tissue-specific stains include:

(a) Safranin O/fast green (paraffin embedding) to confirm a lack of cartilage formation

- Deparaffinize and hydrate sections to water.

- Add 20 μl Weigert's working solution to each section and stain for 30 s to 7 min (depending on age of reagents).

- Wash sections with water for 10 min; change water as necessary.

- Add 20 μl fast green solution to each section and stain for 3 min.

- Immerse sections in 1 % acetic acid for 10–15 s.

- Wash sections with water for 1 min.
- Add 20 μl Safranin O solution to each section and stain for 5 min.
- Dehydrate and clear sections with graded ethanols and xylenes, and then mount in resinous medium.

(b) Von Kossa/MacNeal's tetrachrome (plastic embedding, undecalcified bone) to highlight osteoblast and mineralized bone surfaces

- Deplastify sections and hydrate to water.
- Stain in silver nitrate solution for 10 min in the dark.
- Rinse in distilled water × 3 for 1 min each.
- Stain in sodium carbonate-formaldehyde solution for 2 min.
- Rinse in distilled water × 2 for 1 min each.
- Add potassium ferricyanide to Farmer's diminisher solution. Stain in Farmer's diminisher for 30 s (time is critical).
- Wash in running tap water for 20 min.
- Rinse in distilled water for 1 min.
- Stain in MacNeal's tetrachrome solution for 10–15 min.
- Rinse in distilled water × 3 for 1 min each.
- Dehydrate in one change each of 70 % EtOH, 95 % EtOH, and 100 % EtOH; blot between changes of alcohol.
- Clear in two changes of xylenes.
- Coverslip with xylene-based mounting medium.

(c) Unstained sections (plastic embedding, undecalcified bone) for visualization of fluorochrome labels, if administered (*see* **Note 3**).

3. Quantify osteoblastic histomorphometric indices across the entire defect region via image analysis software [14]. Suggested indices include:

(a) Osteoblast surface/bone surface (Ob.S/BS, %).

(b) Osteoblast number per bone area (N.Ob/B.Ar #/mm^2).

(c) Osteoblast number per tissue area (N.Ob/T.Ar #/mm^2).

4   Notes

1. It can be helpful to replace standard water bottles with ones featuring a long spout, to promote easy access to water without the necessity to rear on hind legs.

2. The most common complication observed from this procedure is the creation of a full femoral fracture. The reported rate of this complication is approximately 4 % (i.e., 1 out of 24 animals [5]). If this occurs, mice should be removed from the study and humanely euthanized. For mice with relatively weak skeletons, reduce cage housing density of the animals to limit the risk of femoral fracture from routine activity.

3. Fluorochrome labeling can be performed prior to tissue harvest to highlight sites of new bone formation. A suggested dosage and administration schedule for calcein has been previously described as 10 mg/kg body mass, injected 10 days after surgery and 4 days prior to animal sacrifice [5].

4. It may be advantageous to harvest and save the contralateral femur, for an intact comparison, or other bones for simultaneous analysis of developmental or systemic phenotypes.

Acknowledgements

The NIH (R01 DE020194, T32 AR056950, F32 AR60140) and the Mayo Clinic Center for Regenerative Medicine supported this work. The authors thank Keith Condon (Indiana University School of Medicine) for the Von Kossa/MacNeal's tetrachrome staining protocol.

References

1. Colnot C (2009) Skeletal cell fate decisions within periosteum and bone marrow during bone regeneration. J Bone Miner Res 24:274–282

2. Morgan EF, Salisbury Palomares KT, Gleason RE et al (2010) Correlations between local strains and tissue phenotypes in an experimental model of skeletal healing. J Biomech 43:2418–2424

3. Le AX, Miclau T, Hu D et al (2001) Molecular aspects of healing in stabilized and non-stabilized fractures. J Orthop Res 19:78–84

4. Cullinane DM, Fredrick A, Eisenberg SR et al (2002) Induction of a neoarthrosis by precisely controlled motion in an experimental mid-femoral defect. J Orthop Res 20:579–586

5. Monfoulet L, Rabier B, Chassande O et al (2010) Drilled hole defects in mouse femur as models of intramembranous cortical and cancellous bone regeneration. Calcif Tissue Int 86:72–81

6. Yu YY, Bahney C, Hu D et al (2012) Creating rigidly stabilized fractures for assessing intra-membranous ossification, distraction osteogenesis, or healing of critical sized defects. J Vis Exp 62, pii:3552

7. Isefuku S, Joyner CJ, Simpson AH (2000) A murine model of distraction osteogenesis. Bone 27:661–665

8. Yan Y, Tang D, Chen M et al (2009) Axin2 controls bone remodeling through the beta-catenin-BMP signaling pathway in adult mice. J Cell Sci 122:3566–3578

9. McGee-Lawrence ME, Ryan ZC, Carpio LR et al (2013) Sclerostin deficient mice rapidly heal bone defects by activating beta-catenin and increasing intramembranous ossification. Biochem Biophys Res Commun 441:886–890

10. Cunliffe-Beamer TL (1993) Applying principles of aseptic surgery to rodents. AWIC Newslett 4:3–6

11. Bouxsein ML, Boyd SK, Christiansen BA et al (2010) Guidelines for assessment of bone microstructure in rodents using micro-computed tomography. J Bone Miner Res 25:1468–1486

12. An YH, Moreira PL, Kang QK et al (2003) Principles of embedding and common protocols. In: An YH, Martin KL (eds) Handbook of histology methods for bone and cartilage. Humana Press, Totowa, NJ, pp 185–206

13. Ries WL (2003) Techniques for sectioning undecalcified bone tissue using microtomes. In: An YH, Martin KL (eds) Handbook of histology methods for bone and cartilage. Humana Press, Totowa, NJ, pp 221–232

14. Dempster DW, Compston JE, Drezner MK et al (2013) Standardized nomenclature, symbols, and units for bone histomorphometry: a 2012 update of the report of the ASBMR Histomorphometry Nomenclature Committee. J Bone Miner Res 28:2–17

Chapter 15

Surgical Procedures and Experimental Outcomes of Closed Fractures in Rodent Models

Hicham Drissi and David N. Paglia

Abstract

The closed fracture rat model, first described by Bonnarens and Einhorn, has been widely implemented in recent years to characterize various fracture phenotypes and evaluate treatment modalities. Slight modifications in the fixation depth, to reduce surgical error associated with movement/dislocation of the k-wire fixation, were previously described. Here, we describe this method which involves the creation of a medial parapatellar incision, dislocation of the patella, boring an 18 gauge hole through the center of the femur, delivery of an adjunct (if applicable), fixation of the k-wire in the greater trochanter of the femur, suturing of muscle and skin, and finally creation of the mid-diaphyseal fracture with a three-point bending fracture device. Many laboratories routinely perform surgical procedures in which a closed fracture is induced using rat or mouse models. The benefits of such surgical models range from general orthopaedic trauma applications to the assessment of the healing process in genetically modified animals. Other important applications include the assessment of the safety and efficacy of various treatment modalities as well as the characterization of bone repair in metabolic bone diseases or skeletal dysplasia.

Key words Closed fractures, Rodent, Surgical procedure, Torsional testing, Histology, Micro-CT

1 Introduction

The use of animals in biomedical research is a privilege. It provides scientists with an invaluable asset, which comes with great responsibility. When conducting survival surgeries using small laboratory animals, researchers must be in compliance with their institutional guidelines (IACUC procedures/guidelines), which reflect state and federal regulations for animal welfare and pain management. We therefore must treat laboratory animals with respect and avoid unnecessary use while ensuring the safety for all involved and the high quality of the data generated. Below we describe closed fracture procedure using rats as experimental models.

Jennifer J. Westendorf and Andre J. van Wijnen (eds.), *Osteoporosis and Osteoarthritis*, Methods in Molecular Biology, vol. 1226, DOI 10.1007/978-1-4939-1619-1_15, © Springer Science+Business Media New York 2015

Bonnarens and Einhorn first described the closed fracture model in 1984 [1]. Since then it has become the standard model for characterization of various fracture phenotypes [2–19]. Widespread acceptance and use of this model has afforded scientists and clinicians alike an invaluable translational model, which is commonly used to examine bone repair under various treatment and pathological conditions.

Following administration of anesthetics, this method involves the creation of a medial parapatellar incision and dislocation of the patella bone, without rupturing the patellar tendon. An 18 gauge needle is used to bore a hole through the midsagittal, mid-coronal plane, above the femoral condyles. Afterwards, an adjunct (if applicable) may be delivered locally. The k-wire is drilled into the greater trochanter of the femur, and the muscle and skin are sutured. Finally, the operated limb of the rat is held perpendicular to the line of fracture, beneath a three-point bending fracture, wherein a transverse fracture is created. Administration of postoperative antibiotics/analgesics reduces the likelihood of infection and helps to manage pain.

To quantify the quality/strength of newly formed bone, micro-CT imaging and torsional testing provide direct measures of fracture healing and bone quality. Bone may be stored in a –20 °C freezer for up to 6 months and covered in saline-soaked gauze prior to testing. Micro-CT scans should be taken the same day as the torsional testing is performed and bones should be wrapped in saline-soaked gauze on ice when not being tested. Radiographic scoring is a useful qualitative measure of fracture healing, which assigns scores characteristic of healing progression.

To evaluate the healing process limbs are typically harvested following euthanasia in a time course that spans a few days to several weeks. Histological assessments allow us to determine the distribution of cartilage, bone, and stroma in the fractured limbs at the site of injury. Typically, specimens are fixed in formalin as needed and processed for histology. Histomorphometric analyses may aid in understanding the progression or delay in fracture healing, while immunohistochemical analyses may be useful in detecting cells/tissues that are positive for growth factors/cytokines involved in fracture healing. Analysis of gene expression from fracture calluses via RT-qPCR provides a temporal relation of gene expression between different experimental models and treatments.

2 Materials

2.1 Closed Fracture Model

1. Personnel: It is optimal to have two researchers involved in this surgery [2–5, 10–12]. The first researcher (assistant) is needed to prepare the animals and manipulate non-sterile objects. The second researcher (surgeon) performs the surgeries under sterile conditions (see Note 1).

2. Anesthetics/analgesics/antibiotics: Ketamine/xylazine (0.9 mL ketamine/0.6 mL xylazine per kilogram body weight), buprenorphine (0.01 mg/kg administered intramuscularly), 3× antibiotic ointment, and Baytril (5–10 mg/kg administered subcutaneously) (*see* **Notes 2** and **3**).

3. Standard surgical equipment: A hemostat, scalpel (preferably size 3, for # 10 blades), #10 blades, forceps, betadine solution, sterile saline solution, resorbable vicryl sutures (size 4-0), 18 gauge needles, wire clippers, gauze, surgical drapes, sterile gloves, an appropriate length of 0.04 in. diameter k-wire (based on the number of surgeries: approx. 40 mm per rat; Small Parts), and a small battery-operated drill (*see* **Note 4**). If an adjunct to augment healing is being administered during the surgery, it should also be available. All surgical equipment should be opened and maintained in a sterile fashion (*see* **Note 5**).

4. Sterile gloves.

5. Radiographic film and cassettes/labels for imaging of the fracture unless digital X-rays are available.

6. A small animal X-ray device for confirmation of the fracture and evaluation of healing.

2.2 Microcomputed Tomography (Micro-CT)

1. Saline-soaked gauze.

2. Portable hard drive to extract data.

3. A micro-CT machine/computer, warmed up for at least 20–30 min.

4. Styrofoam.

5. Set of phantoms (if bone mineral density is being measured).

6. A testing protocol that indicates area of the scan/duration, tube voltage (kVP), current × time product (mAs), and special resolution (µm).

2.3 Torsional Testing

1. Personnel: It is optimal to have two researchers involved during biomechanical testing [2–5]. The first researcher is needed to measure and fixate the samples. The second researcher is needed to test the samples as the first researcher prepares them.

2. Double-boiler filled (*see* **Notes 6** and **7**).

3. Solid Field's metal (or alternative fixatives such as PMMA, Bondo).

4. Wire clippers.

5. Large forceps.

6. Large flathead screwdriver.

7. Appropriately sized square nuts.

8. Stand with a grip to gently hold the epiphysis of the femora.

9. Sterile saline solution.

10. Gauze.

11. Camera.

12. Labels for pictures.

13. Caliper for measurements.

14. Nitrile gloves.

15. Goggles.

16. Waterproof marker.

17. Material of known strength that is used for machine calibration (if applicable).

18. Mechanical testing apparatus/computer with a load cell which is sensitive enough to detect sample differences in the order or 0.5–5 N mm with appropriate tools to manipulate the machine (*see* **Note 8**). The samples should be maintained and experimental equipment set up appropriately (*see* **Notes 9–11**).

2.4 Radiographic Scoring

1. Personnel: It is necessary to have two independent observers, trained to evaluate X-rays [3], score radiographs. It is optimal to have a separate researcher blind radiographs for analysis and analyze data.

2. Anteroposterior (AP) and lateral radiographs from successful (transverse mid-diaphyseal fracture) surgical procedures (usually scored from radiographs at 2–4 weeks after fracture at earliest) which the observers cannot associate with any particular experimental group.

3. Sheets labeled for observers to fill out with scoring scales and coded sample numbers.

4. Software for appropriate data analysis.

5. AP and lateral radiographs, coded to avoid association with experimental groups.

6. Scoring criteria and assessment sheets.

2.5 Histology

1. Paraffin embedding: Formalin, an orbital shaker, a chelator such as EDTA solution (pH 6.9–7.1) for decalcification of experimental specimens, 70, 80, 95, and 100 % ETOH, xylene, paraffin wax, a vacuum oven, a fume hood, razor blades, metal molds for embedding, embedding cassettes, and an embedding center to make paraffin blocks,

2. Paraffin sectioning: Freezer, paraffin blocks to be sectioned, a microtome capable of cutting sections as thin as 5 μm, a hot water bath (42–48 °C), slides, a rack for drying of slides.

3. PMMA embedding: Formalin, an orbital shaker, 70, 80, 95, and 100 % ETOH, xylene, PMMA (I, II, and III), small glass bottles with lids, freezer bags, plastic sample collection bags,

small aluminum caps used for embedding, a fume hood, scissors, hammer, a water bath, and a refrigerator kept at 4 °C (*see* **Notes 12–15**).

4. PMMA sectioning: Saw with a diamond-tipped blade, aluminum foil, 100 % ETOH, a polishing wheel, polishing disk, PMMA-embedding glue, and slides.

5. Staining materials: Containers filled with 70, 95, and 100 % ETOH, xylene, distilled water, cover slips, and appropriate mounting solution.

6. Immunohistochemistry materials: 1× TBST (100 ml 10× Tris-buffered saline (TBS) combined with 900 ml deionized water), a blocking buffer (5 ml 1× TBST combined with 250 μl normal goat serum), a temperature-controlled steamer capable of reaching 100 °C, a fluorescence microscope, an appropriate antigen retrieval solution (e.g., sodium citrate), and appropriate diluted primary/conjugated secondary antibodies (*see* **Note 16**).

7. Histomorphometric quantification: Appropriate analysis software, microscope with camera, a small surgical ruler or scale slide for image dimensional calibration, and a statistical analyses software.

2.6 RT-PCR

1. Cryogenic tissue homogenizer or alternatively a mortar and pestle.

2. Surgical tool to separate bone.

3. Liquid nitrogen.

4. Aluminum foil.

5. TRIzol solution.

6. Microcentrifuge tubes.

7. Chloroform.

8. Temperature-controlled centrifuge.

9. RNase-free glycogen.

10. 100 % isopropanol.

11. 75 % ethanol.

12. UV spectrophotometer or NanoDrop machine.

13. RNA reverse transcription kit (e.g., iScriptTM cDNA Synthesis Kit) (*see* **Note 17**).

14. Thermal cycler.

15. Computer and real-time PCR machine [e.g., Biosystems 7500 Real-Time PCR System (Applied Biosystems, Foster City, CA)].

16. RNase/DNase-free water.

17. Forward and reverse primers for genes of interest and house-keeping gene (e.g., β-actin, GAPDH) (*see* **Note 17**).

18. PCR plates and covers compatible with PCR machine.

19. Centrifuge with plate holder attachments.

3   Methods

3.1   Closed Fracture Model

Surgeries should be performed in a clean, surgical suite on a surface wiped down with 70 % ethanol.

1. Assuming a standard unilateral surgery, administer a cocktail of ketamine/xylazine to the rat (*see* **Note 18**).

2. Once unresponsive to stimuli, shave the entire surgical leg and adjacent skin well and coat with betadine solution.

3. After the solution is dried, clean the surgical site with sterile saline solution.

4. Cut drapes to expose a hole only large enough to slip the surgical limb through.

5. Once isolated, the surgeon holds the operated limb with the middle finger positioned underneath the knee and the index finger resting on the quadriceps muscle. The thumb is held against the tibia for balance.

6. Using their other hand, the surgeon creates a medial parapatellar incision through the skin and muscle until contact with the femur is detected. The quadriceps muscle is dislocated and the femoral condyles are exposed, being careful to avoid any contact with the patellar tendon (Fig. 1a).

7. Position the 18 gauge needle to midsagittal, mid-coronal (*see* **Note 19**), directly above the condyles (*see* **Note 20**) and rotate gently (without applying pressure) in a single direction until the marrow cavity is punctured (*see* **Note 21**). The marrow cavity is exposed. Rinse it with sterile saline.

8. The assistant surgeon positions the drill and loads it with k-wire of an appropriate length (40–50 mm). Set the drill to its lowest setting and run it until the k-wire punctures the marrow space into the greater trochanter (*see* **Note 22**).

9. Relocate the quadriceps muscle and suture the adjacent muscle to the patellar tendon using a running stitch. Tie appropriately.

10. Suture the skin using interrupted mattress sutures to ensure that the rats do not bite open the wound after recovery.

11. Position the rat on its back with the diaphysis of its femur perpendicular to the blunt lower guillotine blade (Fig. 1b). The assistant applies a preload force, until the femur is locked

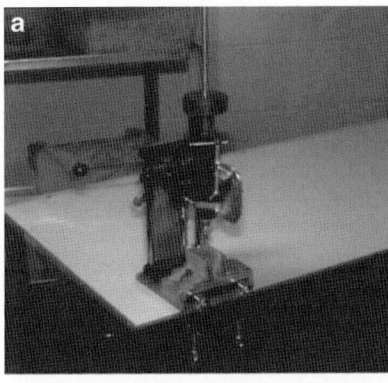 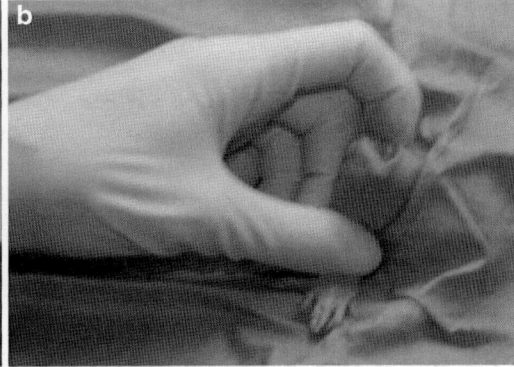

Fig. 1 Rodent undergoing a standard closed femoral fracture procedure. (**a**) Three-point bending fracture device, (**b**) exposure of the femoral condyle prior to boring through the condyle trabecular bone

in the desired position and then drops a 250–500 g weight from a predetermined height (typically 10–35 cm), to induce a high-energy fracture (*see* **Note 23**).

12. Take an X-ray to confirm the fracture. Then administer buprenorphine for pain management (*see* **Note 24**), and Baytril/3× ointment antibiotics once daily for the first 2 days post-op.

13. Take radiographs at 1–2-week intervals to ensure the fixation of the k-wire and track healing.

14. Monitor rats for the first 3 days to ensure that they bear weight on their operated limb.

3.2 MicroCT Scanning

1. Defrost bones in a lukewarm water bath for 30–40 min and place on ice.

2. Verify the pre-programmed testing conditions (*see* **Note 25**).

3. Place styrofoam around the bone(s) being tested and insert it along with the appropriate phantom (if applicable) in the machine attachment that will be docked.

4. Dock the attachment and the close machine.

5. Select the areas of interest and analysis program. The machine computes the estimated completion time of the scan.

6. Start the scan and wait for the indicated time until the next sample(s) may be processed.

7. Repeat **steps 3–6** until all the samples are scanned.

8. Reconstruct scan (Fig. 2) and extract for further analysis (*see* **Note 26**).

9. Turn the machine off.

10. Images are then segmented (and a global threshold is applied if applicable) and analyzed.

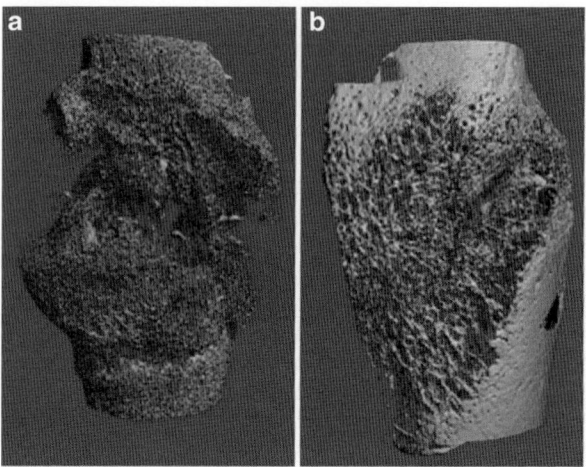

Fig. 2 Examples of micro-CT reconstructions for rodent fracture calluses at (**a**) 14 days post-fracture, (**b**) 21 days post-fracture

3.3   Torsional Testing   Whenever biomechanical testing is performed care must be taken to ensure the safety of both the individual performing the test and those in the surrounding area. Many machines, including those used for testing of smaller samples, must be operated carefully and testing protocols should be programmed with emergency shut-down conditions (Fig. 3a).

1. Defrost bone in a lukewarm water bath for 30–40 min and place on ice.

2. The double-boiler should be half-filled with water and set to reach boiling temperature.

3. Turn on the mechanical testing apparatus with load cell attached.

4. Remove any remaining tissue carefully using dry gauze. Slowly and carefully pull the surgical k-wire from the fractured femora (*see* **Note 27**). Rewrap the bones in saline-soaked gauze and place on ice (*see* **Note 28**).

5. Measure the total length, maximum outer diameter within the diaphyseal region, and minimum outer diameter within the diaphyseal region of the femora with a caliper and record.

6. Take pictures of all bones before testing and label as "before failure" pictures (Fig. 3b, c).

7. Fix each femur by firmly positioning its extremities in the stand/holder above one of the square nuts with the femoral condyles positioned inside the nut (*see* **Note 29**). Pour the fixative (i.e., Field's metal) within the nut to cement each extremity (*see* **Note 30**). Allow it to solidify for approximately 5 min. Rotate the femur in the stand/holder and the head/

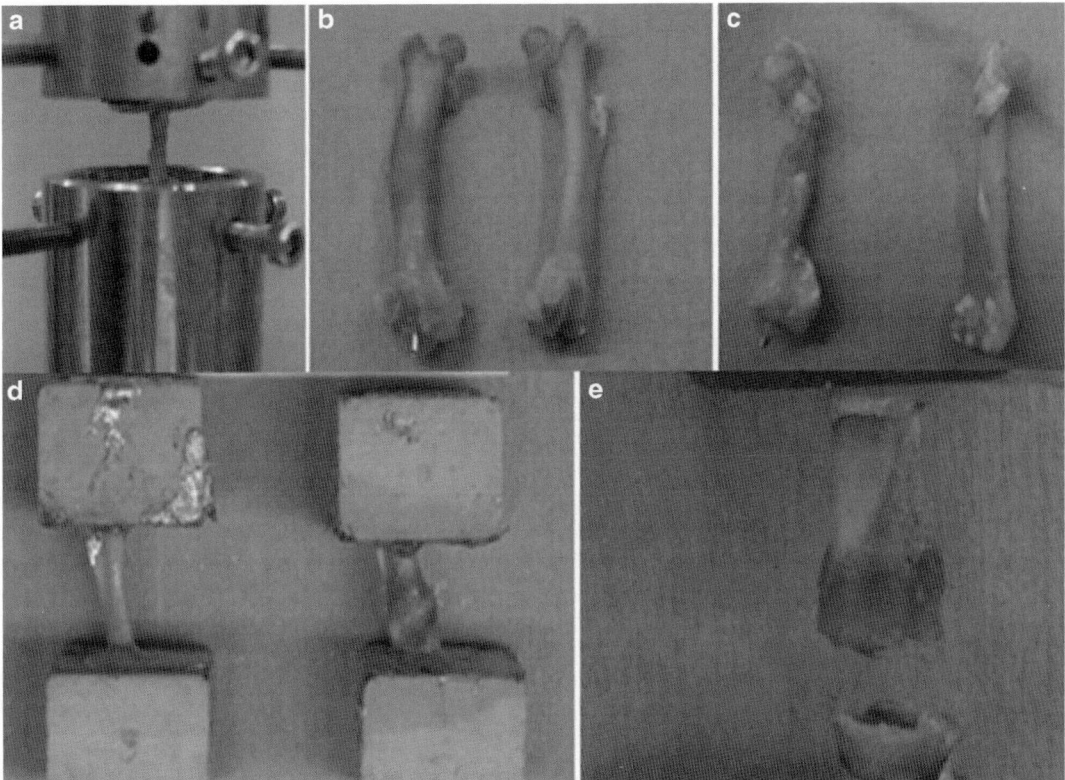

Fig. 3 Torsional testing of rat femora. (**a**) Torsional testing setup, (**b** and **c**) femora prior to potting, (**d**) fractured and contralateral femora after potting in low-temperature metal, (**e**) fractured femur after torsional testing to yield

greater trochanter of the femur should be embedded in the fixative. Allow the Field's metal to dry for another 5 min. Measure and record gauge length for all specimens (*see* **Note 31**). Take pictures to confirm sample alignment (Fig. 3d).

8. As one researcher continues to fixate specimens, the other may setup and calibrate the testing apparatus. All the default machine forces/torques/positions should be reset as should the interlocks (if applicable). The investigator should ensure that all testing hardware is appropriately attached, including the load cell.

9. Start and configure the software for the calibration. The testing outputs/data analysis should be set (if applicable).

10. Place the first specimen in the testing apparatus and tighten one (i.e., fixated nut) end into place. Remove the gauze around the bone and record the torque as "zeroed."

11. Being careful not to damage the specimen, slowly tighten (pre-torque up to 20 N mm for rat bones) the second end until locked. After the position is set, zero the torque and run the

test. Record inner and outer maximum diaphyseal diameters for all samples after testing. Take pictures to confirm the fracture failure mode (Fig. 3e).

12. Repeat this procedure for all samples.

13. Turn off all machinery and the double boiler.

14. Extract the data and analyze the torque curves to verify testing accuracy.

3.4 Radiographic Scoring

1. Code and shuffle the radiographs (*see* **Note 32**) of appropriate fractures (Fig. 4a) to avoid any experimental group association (*see* **Note 33**).

2. Instruct observers to evaluate AP and lateral radiographs (*see* **Note 34**) according to the following criteria:

   The analysis should be conducted in a blinded fashion using a validated radiographic scoring system, subdivided into the following categories: (a) periosteal and endosteal reaction, (b) callus opacity, and (c) cortical remodeling and bridging (Fig. 4b).

   (a) The periosteal and endosteal bridging is determined using a four-point scoring system, 0 = no reaction, 1 = mild reaction, 2 = moderate reaction, and 3 = marked reaction (bridging across the osteotomy).

   (b) The callus opacity bridging is determined using a four-point scoring system, 0 = no evidence of mineralization, 1 = heterogeneous with minimal mineralization and cortices well demarcated, 2 = heterogeneous with moderate mineralization and partially confluent with the cortices, and 3 = confluent with the cortices, uniform (Fig. 4b).

   (c) Finally, the cortical remodeling and bridging are determined using a five-point scoring system, 0 = no apparent remodeling, 1 = all cortical edges seen but ill defined, 2 = minimal cortical union (three cortical edges visible) without reformation of the medullary canal, 3 = partial cortical union (1–2 cortical edges visible) with visible

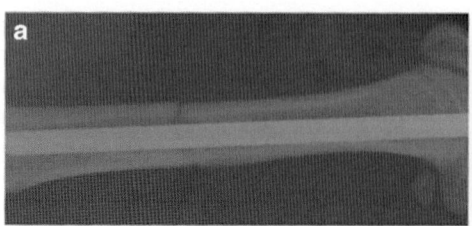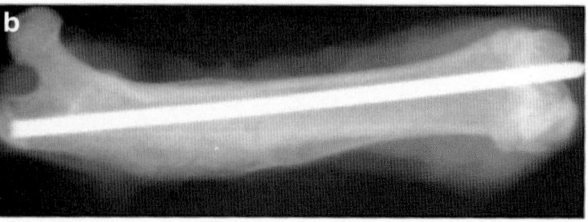

Fig. 4 Radiographic images. (**a**) Acceptable fracture pattern following surgery, (**b**) fractured femora representative of fully bridged, headed bone (total score = 10)

medullary canal, and 4 = complete cortical union (no cortical edges visible) with well-demarcated medullary canal.

3. Collect evaluation sheet and perform appropriate statistical analyses.

3.5 Histology

The methodology outlined below describes general procedures for histological fixation, sample preparation, sectioning, and histomorphometric quantification. Due to the wide variety of staining procedures/conditions, the experimenter is advised to consult online literature/publications relevant to the staining procedures needed to visualize specific tissue components. It is essential that the researcher remains consistent with all procedures to allow better comparative analyses.

3.5.1 Paraffin Embedding

1. Immediately after rodent euthanasia, collect operative limbs and strip off excessive soft tissue (there should be some soft tissue remaining to maintain structural integrity of the fractured bones).

2. Fix bones in 4 % formalin on an orbital shaker at room temperature for about 2 weeks (*see* **Note 35**).

3. Rinse fixed bones under running water for 30 min (*see* **Note 36**).

4. Place bones in embedding cassettes in the presence of a chelator for 2–3 weeks to decalcify.

5. Once bones are somewhat pliable (7–10 days after decalcification), cut one side of each femur (with soft tissue) flat with a razor blade so that the bone surface is slightly exposed, without compromising the fracture site.

6. Rinse decalcified bones under running water for 30 min.

7. Place cassettes in 70 % ETOH for 2 h, 80 % ETOH for 2 h, 95 % ETOH for 2 h, three separate 100 % ETOH solutions for 2 h each, three separate xylene solutions for 2 h each, two separate heated liquid paraffin solutions for 2 h each, and paraffin solution in a heated vacuum oven for 1 h.

8. Remove bones from cassettes and carefully retrieve the intramedullary pin from each fractured femur.

9. Embed bones in hot paraffin wax (with flat side which was cut during decalcification facing down, positioned in the center of a metallic mold) on an embedding center and allow them to cool on the appropriate station.

10. Solidify the wax gradually, by popping the air bubbles that form in the center of the wax mold.

11. Label the samples and allow them to cool on the embedding station for 2 h before storing them at –20 °C.

3.5.2 Paraffin Sectioning

1. Label all slides for specimen collection.
2. Turn on the hot water bath 30 min before sectioning (set on 5 μm thin sections).
3. Place a sharp sectioning blade in the microtome.
4. Remove paraffin blocks from the –20 °C freezer (placed beneath ice), and move it near to the microtome (*see* **Note 37**).
5. Carefully position each block in the microtome and coarsely section (25 μm) until the tissue sample is exposed.
6. Place the block beneath ice for 10–20 min.
7. Section the block at a setting of 5–7 μm, creating ribbons.
8. Carefully place ribbons on surface of the water in the water bath.
9. Allow paraffin ribbon sections to stand for 1–2 min in the bath, before being carefully placed onto appropriate slides.
10. Leave slides overnight to dry on the slide-drying rack.
11. Repeat this procedure until the sample is fully sectioned.

3.5.3 PMMA Embedding

1. Place fixed bones (same fixation procedure as for paraffin embedding) in 70 % ETOH for 1 day.
2. Transfer to 80 % ETOH for 1 day.
3. Transfer to 95 % ETOH for 1 day.
4. Transfer to 100 % ETOH solutions for 1 day.
5. Repeat **step 4** two times.
6. Transfer to xylene for 1 day.
7. Repeat **step 6** two times.
8. Transfer to PMMA I for 3 days (*see* **Note 38**).
9. Transfer specimens to covered glass jars after positioning them inside cut metal-embedding caps.
10. Place specimens in PMMA II solution and allow them to rock on the orbital shaker for 4 h, before returning them to the refrigerator in PMMA II solution.
11. Repeat **step 10** daily for 3 days.
12. Place specimens in a third PMMA III solution following the same procedure as for PMMA II.
13. Store bottles in a warm water bath for 3 days.
14. Upon solidification of PMMA III, place bottles in freezer bags and carefully crack them with a hammer under the hood.
15. Clean blocks of excess glass and rinse them with deionized water.
16. Label blocks and place them within sealed sample bags.
17. Store sample bags in a sealed container, away from open air.

3.5.4 PMMA Sectioning

1. Label all slides for tissue collection.

2. Set up a saw with aluminum foil shielding the area adjacent to the blade.

3. Supply the blade with a constant stream of 100 % ETOH (diamond saws are usually set up for this).

4. Cut blocks with the saw (diamond tip blade) to expose the surface to be sectioned.

5. Section PMMA blocks at the desired thickness.

6. Polish sections on a polisher with a rotating polishing wheel (with polishing disk).

7. Mount sections to slides with glue.

3.5.5 Histological/IHC Staining

1. Rehydrate slides (generally 10 min in xylene, 5 min in xylene, 2 min in 100 % ETOH, 2 min in 100 % ETOH, 2 min in 95 % ETOH, 2 min in 70 % ETOH, 2 min in 50 % ETOH, 2 min in deionized water).

2. Conduct histological staining/IHC procedure (differs depending on experiment: consult online literature) on rehydrated slides (*see* **Note 39**). Slides may need to be dehydrated and placed in xylene after staining for some protocols.

3. Cover slip slides and allow them to dry under aluminum foil at room temperature overnight.

3.5.6 Histomorphometric Quantification

1. Visualized slides under appropriate microscope magnification (different analyses require different fields of view) and capture pictures with camera software.

2. Capture a 1-mm-scale picture at the same magnification when taking these pictures.

3. Use software such as ImageJ, ImagePro, and Osteomeasure for image analyses. Different analyses may require different software (consult chosen software documentation for more details). Mineralized tissue/fibrous tissue/cartilage matrix can be quantified, and normalized to the total callus area. Total number of cells and cells expressing certain factors can be counted (*see* **Note 40**) and their total normalized to the area of analyses (*see* **Note 41**).

4. Analyze data using appropriate statistical approaches.

3.6 RT-PCR

Whenever qRT-PCR is performed care must be taken to ensure that solutions are not contaminated with RNases/DNases. Careful laboratory practices should be upheld to support the validity of any data generated.

1. Isolate fracture calluses within 2 min of animal euthanasia and flash freeze them in liquid nitrogen after removing all surrounding soft tissue, pulling out the pin, carefully excising the

surrounding bone from the intact fracture callus (calluses should be placed in labeled aluminum foil pouches, immediately before freezing).

2. Store frozen bones in foil pouches in a –80 °C freezer for further processing.

3. Homogenize calluses into a fine powder using either a tissue homogenizer or a mortar and pestle, maintained at –80 °C.

4. Dissolve homogenized samples in an appropriate volume of TRIzol (in microcentrifuge tubes) and allow samples to incubate for 5 min at room temperature.

5. Add 0.2 mL of chloroform per 1 mL TRIzol reagent to the samples and shake tubes vigorously by hand for 15 s.

6. Incubate samples at room temperature for 2–3 min and subsequently centrifuge them at $12,000 \times g$ for 15 min at 4 °C.

7. Isolate the aqueous phase (*see* **Note 42**) and pipette it into a new tube with 5–10 μg of RNase-free glycogen and 0.5 mL of 100 % isopropanol per 1 mL TRIzol used.

8. Incubate the mixture at room temperature for 10 min and subsequently centrifuge it at $12,000 \times g$ for 10 min at 4 °C.

9. Remove the supernatant from the tube, leaving only the RNA pellet, which is washed in 1 mL 75 % ethanol per 1 mL TRIzol used.

10. Briefly vortex the mixture and centrifuge at $7,500 \times g$ for 5 min at 4 °C.

11. Discard the ethanol wash and air-dry the pellet for 10–15 min (without drying out the RNA pellet completely).

12. Resuspend the RNA pellet in 7–10 μl of RNase-free water or 0.5 % SDS.

13. Incubate the RNA-water suspensions in a heat bath set at 55–60 °C for 10–15 min.

14. Store them at –80 °C for downstream applications.

15. After the RNA is defrosted in an ice bucket, determine RNA content via Nanodrop readings/UV spectrometer.

16. Dilute the RNA aliquots in RNase-free water to ensure that all samples have the same concentration of RNA.

17. Reverse transcribe the RNA according to the kit/procedure used (using a thermal cycler (if available)). cDNA obtained from reverse transcription can be refrigerated at –20 °C with forward and reverse primer stock.

18. Prepare primer and cDNA cocktails for all genes of interest and housekeeping genes, ensuring that each tube has the same concentration of forward primer, reverse primer, cDNA cocktail, and SYBR green mix (if SYBR green is used) for a total of 10 μL (*see* **Note 43**).

19. Spin tubes briefly to remove bubbles.

20. Pipette 10 μL of solution into a new set of PCR tubes (corresponding to the eventual RT-PCR plates). There should be three replicates per tube of cDNA/primer cocktail.

21. Spin tubes briefly to remove bubbles.

22. Set up an ice bath with the RT-PCR plate and PCR tubes.

23. Transfer the contents of the PCR plates into the wells.

24. Cover the plate with plastic tightly and centrifuge the plate held in place by a plate holder.

25. Input samples in a compatible plate into the thermal cycler and set the machine for PCR analysis. Add labels to the program and run standard PCR according to appropriate conditions for the sample of interest.

26. Record Ct values and input them into an excel spreadsheet for data analysis.

27. Perform data analysis for obtained CT values, relating expression of genes of interest to housekeeping genes (*see* **Note 44**).

4   Notes

1. Although the use of rats is described in this protocol, this procedure may be performed on mice (useful when examining transgenic models). The size of the fracture device/weight dropped, size of the needle/sutures/surgical blade/k-wire must all be adjusted for the mouse model and the drill is not necessary.

2. It is optimal to prepare all anesthetic cocktails before surgery has begun.

3. If they resist the anesthetics, rodents may be continuously administered small doses of isoflurane upon IACUC approval.

4. Before performing this procedure, it is useful that the surgeon practices dislocation of the quadriceps muscle and patellar bone on "practice" animals.

5. All metallic equipment (except for the drill) and the surgical tray(s) should be cleansed with enzymatic detergent prior to any surgery. All metallic equipment (except for the drill), gauze, and drapes should be wrapped in surgical drapes and autoclaved (using a standard cycle) to sterilize them prior to surgery. Blades, needles, sutures, and saline should be opened in a sterile fashion over the opened sterilized surgical tray. The drill should be rubbed down in betadine and allowed to dry on a sterile surface, adjacent to the surgical tray.

6. The double boiler should be half-filled with water and the water level should be monitored throughout testing.

7. The double boiler should be heated for 20–30 min, set at boiling temperature before use.

8. The mechanical testing apparatus should be allowed to run for at least 1 h before it is used for testing.

9. Fixated bones should be allowed to solidify in Field's metal for 5 min before they are removed from the holder.

10. Bones should be kept in chilled saline-soaked gauze throughout all procedures (except for while the test is running).

11. All specimens should be supported in an unstressed position when moved.

12. All materials should be prepared prior to initiating histological procedures.

13. ETOH at various concentrations can be diluted from 100 % ETOH combined with deionized water.

14. All operations involving formalin, ETOH, xylene, PMMA, and mounting media should be conducted inside a fume hood that is not vented into the workspace.

15. PMMA embedding is advantageous when the researcher is interested in mineralized tissue formation, independent of EDTA decalcification. Disadvantages of PMMA embedding include thick sections, which are generally suboptimal for cellular evaluations and may also limit staining options.

16. Different staining procedures require different materials, dyes, and incubation times. To determine if additional materials are needed and to familiarize the researcher with each specific staining procedure, it is recommended to consult literature online before undertaking an experiment.

17. Reagents should be stored at the appropriate temperatures indicated on the vendors' instructions.

18. If additional anesthetics are needed and rats become sensitized, up to 1/2 of the original dose may be used.

19. When using mice, one can minimize morbidity by punching a hole directly through the skin in the femoral condyle using a 24 G needle. The k-wire is then inserted into the medullary canal and locked via bending of the external extremity and its dissemination under the skin prior to fracturing.

20. For tibia fracture procedures the hole is induced in the tibial plateau to insert the stabilizing pin (k-wire) and the procedure is the same as for the femurs.

21. It is important not to apply excessive pressure when boring through the bone with the needle or when operating the drill to avoid unwanted bone damage.

22. The k-wire is drilled into the greater trochanter to ensure that it will not be dislodged from the intramedullary space after surgery.

23. When investigating mechanisms of bone repair processes associated with microdamage, alternative methods of injury induction must be applied [20, 21].

24. Analgesics can also be administered preoperatively, but any drug administration needs to be preapproved in the animal protocol.

25. It is recommended to scan ex vivo samples with the following parameters: 5 μm resolution, 50 kV tube voltage, and tube current 200 μA, with an in-plane special resolution of 48 μm × 48 μm, but scan parameters can change depending on the particular experiment [10, 11].

26. In vivo micro-CT scanning must take into account soft tissue and may use a contrast medium.

27. It is useful to brace the second fixated end as it is slowly tightened to ensure minimal effects on the pre-torque of the sample being tested.

28. The diaphyseal region of femur should be maintained in cold saline-soaked gauze throughout fixation and testing processes to preserve biomechanical properties and help brace the bone during testing setup.

29. It is useful to embed wooden dowels around the specimen during fixation to reduce stress on the bone prior to testing, but these must be severed before testing to ensure that they do not interfere with testing values.

30. There are several alternatives to potting specimens with low-temperature metal. Common examples include acrylic polymethylmethacrylate (PMMA) and Bondo®. PMMA is hardened through an exothermic reaction wherein a liquid methylmethycrylate monomer (should not exceed three times the volume of the potted specimen region) is added to a polymer powder. In contrast, Bondo® (polyester resin sold in kits) forms moldable putty when mixed with a hardener, which subsequently sets and hardens into a solid geometry.

31. Gauge lengths of all specimens should be within 1.5 mm of each other.

32. The same equipment and settings for X-ray imaging are necessary to perform any semiquantitative analyses across the experimental groups.

33. It is generally acceptable to have either orthopaedic surgeons or experienced orthopaedic researchers who are familiar with the scoring scale participate as observers for radiographic evaluation.

34. Researchers should ensure that group associations remain coded throughout the evaluation process and that they do not introduce any external bias.

35. Frozen embedding may be performed by incubating samples overnight in a 30 % sucrose solution (after formalin fixation) and flash freezing in optimal cutting temperature tissue (OCT) media (within plastic cassettes) surrounded by either liquid nitrogen or an alternative (e.g., dry ice and 100 % ethanol).

36. A pencil should be used for marking all histological containers/cassettes.

37. Frozen sectioning may be performed using OCT medium for sample mounting and a Cryostat for sample sectioning.

38. Samples should always be kept on the orbital shaker when solutions are not being changed.

39. IHC primary antibody dilutions should be verified in the researcher's lab with positive and negative controls, as well as with femoral tissue samples, prior to any IHC staining.

40. There are different techniques for quantifying the number of cells after IHC staining. Some studies set a baseline level of staining intensity and count positive cells above that level. Other studies count all cells with moderate staining and above.

41. Some recent studies [3, 4] found statistically significant cellular differences in the subperiosteal region of the fracture callus within the first 2 weeks of healing. Segmentation of counts within separate regions of the callus may yield interesting results, outlining the importance of the periosteum in fracture healing [22, 23].

42. The interphase and organic phenol chloroform can be stored at 4 °C overnight if isolation of DNA or protein is desired.

43. All primers should be validated prior to interpretation and publication of data.

44. The RT-PCR conditions should be optimized to obtain appropriate melt curves.

References

1. Bonnarens F, Einhorn TA (1984) Production of a standard closed fracture in laboratory animal bone. J Orthop Res 2:97–101

2. Paglia DN, Wey A, Vaidya S et al (2013) Effects of local insulin delivery on subperiosteal angiogenesis and mineralized tissue formation during fracture healing. J Orthop Res 31:783–791

3. Park AG, Paglia DN, Al-Zube L et al (2013) Local insulin therapy affects fracture healing in a rat model. J Orthop Res 31:776–782

4. Paglia DN, Wey A, Park AG et al (2012) The effects of local vanadium treatment on angiogenesis and chondrogenesis during fracture healing. J Orthop Res 30:1971–1978

5. Bergenstock M, Min W, Simon AM et al (2005) A comparison between the effects of acetaminophen and celecoxib on bone fracture healing in rats. J Orthop Trauma 19:717–723

6. Schmidmaier G, Wildemann B, Gabelein T et al (2003) Synergistic effect of IGF-I and TGF-beta1 on fracture healing in rats: single versus combined application of IGF-I and TGF-beta1. Acta Orthop Scand 74:604–610

7. Schmidmaier G, Wildemann B, Ostapowicz D et al (2004) Long-term effects of local growth factor (IGF-I and TGF-beta 1) treatment on fracture healing. A safety study for using growth factors. J Orthop Res 22:514–519

8. Kayal RA, Tsatsas D, Bauer MA et al (2007) Diminished bone formation during diabetic fracture healing is related to the premature resorption of cartilage associated with increased osteoclast activity. J Bone Miner Res 22:560–568

9. Kayal RA, Alblowi J, McKenzie E et al (2009) Diabetes causes the accelerated loss of cartilage during fracture repair which is reversed by insulin treatment. Bone 44:357–363

10. Soung DY, Talebian L, Matheny CJ et al (2012) Runx1 dose-dependently regulates endochondral ossification during skeletal development and fracture healing. J Bone Miner Res 27:1585–1597

11. Soung DY, Gentile MA, Duong LT et al (2013) Effects of pharmacological inhibition of cathepsin K on fracture repair in mice. Bone 55:248–255

12. Clifton K, Soung DY, Gibson J et al (2012) Gene array analyses reveal distinct expression patterns in the osteoclast and chondroclast populations within a fracture callus. ASBMR 2012 annual meeting, Minneapolis, MN. Presentation Number: LB-MO13

13. Gerstenfeld LC, Einhorn TA (2003) Developmental aspects of fracture healing and the use of pharmacological agents to alter healing. J Musculoskelet Neuronal Interact 3:297–303

14. Gandhi A, Beam HA, O'Connor JP et al (2005) The effects of local insulin delivery on diabetic fracture healing. Bone 37:482–490

15. Carofino BC, Lieberman JR (2008) Gene therapy applications for fracture-healing. J Bone Joint Surg Am 90:99–110

16. Takahata M, Awad HA, O'Keefe RJ et al (2012) Endogenous tissue engineering: PTH therapy for skeletal repair. Cell Tissue Res 347:545–552

17. Graves DT, Alblowi J, Paglia DN et al (2011) Impact of diabetes on fracture healing. J Exp Clin Med 3:3–8

18. Wu X, Chen S, He Y et al (2011) The haploinsufficient hematopoietic microenvironment is critical to the pathological fracture repair in murine models of neurofibromatosis type 1. PLoS One 6:e24917

19. Gerstenfeld LC, Cullinane DM, Barnes GL et al (2003) Fracture healing as a post-natal developmental process: molecular, spatial, and temporal aspects of its regulation. J Cell Biochem 88:873–884

20. Tami AE, Nasser P, Schaffler MB et al (2003) Noninvasive fatigue fracture model of the rat ulna. J Orthop Res 21:1018–1024

21. Schaffler MB, Kennedy OD (2012) Osteocyte signaling in bone. Curr Osteoporos Rep 10:118–125

22. Zhang X, Awad HA, O'Keefe RJ et al (2008) A perspective: engineering periosteum for structural bone graft healing. Clin Orthop Relat Res 466:1777–1787

23. Balaburski G, O'Connor JP (2003) Determination of variations in gene expression during fracture healing. Acta Orthop Scand 74:22–30

INDEX